Praise for Real Skills for Real Life

"Being a person is painful. Like a good friend, this clear, warm, lively book takes you by the hand and imparts astonishing wisdom and strategies for making it hurt less. *Real Skills for Real Life* is a revelation."

—Jean G., Hudson, New York

"Drs. Rizvi and Finkelstein take skills from DBT and translate them into a salve for daily living. The book explains what skill to use when, how you can tell if it is working, and alternative skills for when it is not. Lively, clever images practically make the skills jump off the page."

—Jill H. Rathus, PhD, Department of Psychology, Long Island University Post; Cognitive Behavioral Associates, Great Neck, New York

"This book gave me the practical tools and guidance I badly needed to drop some behaviors based in fear and shame that have been holding me back for decades—and start making choices that serve me better. I feel like I am breaking free of self-inflicted shackles!"

—Louis S., Woodstock, New York

"Drs. Rizvi and Finkelstein have written a DBT guide for everyone! Clear examples and immersive graphics help you practice these evidence-based skills in real life—even in situations that feel impossible—so you can struggle less and become more resilient."

—Blaise Aguirre, MD, author of *I Hate Myself: Overcome Self-Loathing and Realize Why You're Wrong About You*

"I have spent more than a decade in traditional talk therapy, replaying the same anxious thought loops and intrusive thoughts with only minuscule mood shifts to show for it. This book lays out concrete skills and strategies for navigating life's inevitable ups and downs, helping me to rethink my own emotional resting posture and, if only for intervals, snap out of it. I feel more progress after one read on the sofa than I do after 10 years on the couch."

—Sam C., New York City

"What a gem of a book! Drs. Rizvi and Finkelstein have distilled 26 DBT skills into bite-sized chunks with wonderful illustrations and graphics. I really like the flowcharts that direct you to appropriate skills to try for common challenges. This book will be of use to any human struggling with stresses and crises of any scale, regardless of your background in DBT."

—Michaela A. Swales, PhD, Professor and Program Director, North Wales Clinical Psychology Program, Bangor University, United Kingdom

"DBT offers such a rich, creative, varied approach to problems large and small, and Drs. Rizvi and Finkelstein give you step-by-step tools to put DBT concepts into practice. I know this book will be very helpful when I need an on-the-spot resource to manage anxiety or self-judgment, for example, or prepare for difficult conversations. The visual aids and illustrations make the book approachable and fun. I will definitely recommend and share this resource with many friends in the years ahead."

—Jan D., Woodstock, New York

REAL SKILLS FOR REAL LIFE

Also Available for Professionals

Chain Analysis in Dialectical Behavior Therapy
Shireen L. Rizvi

Dialectical Behavior Therapy in Clinical Practice:
Applications across Disorders and Settings, Second Edition
Edited by Linda A. Dimeff, Shireen L. Rizvi, and Kelly Koerner

REAL SKILLS FOR REAL LIFE

A DBT Guide to Navigating Stress, Emotions, and Relationships

SHIREEN L. RIZVI, PhD
JESSE FINKELSTEIN, PsyD

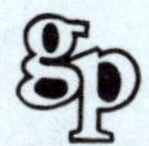

THE GUILFORD PRESS
New York London

A Division of Guilford Publications, Inc.
www.guilford.com

Printed in the United States of America

For product and safety concerns within the EU, please contact *GPSR@taylorandfrancis.com,* Taylor & Francis Verlag GmbH, Kaufingerstraße 24, 80331 München, Germany.

Last digit is print number: 9 8 7 6 5 4 3 2 1

Library of Congress Cataloging-in-Publication Data

Names: Rizvi, Shireen L. author | Finkelstein, Jesse author
Title: Real skills for real life : a DBT guide to navigating stress, emotions, and relationships / Shireen L. Rizvi, PhD, ABPP, Jesse Finkelstein, PsyD.
Description: New York : The Guilford Press, [2026] | Includes index.
Identifiers: LCCN 2025030210 | ISBN 9781462555574 paperback | ISBN 9781462558773 hardcover
Subjects: LCSH: Dialectical behavior therapy | Life skills—Handbooks, manuals, etc. | Stress management
Classification: LCC RC489.D48 R585 2026
LC record available at *https://lccn.loc.gov/2025030210*

CONTENTS

ACKNOWLEDGMENTS

This book has been a labor of love, nearly five years in the making, and we have numerous individuals to thank for helping us bring it to fruition.

We extend our heartfelt gratitude to our mentors, clients, and students, all of whom have played a vital role in shaping us into the Dialectical Behavior Therapy (DBT) clinicians and educators we are today. In particular, we wish to acknowledge Marsha Linehan, whose mentorship profoundly influenced Shireen. Marsha, we are deeply grateful for the skills you have created—these tools have saved countless lives, and we are honored to share them with as many people as possible.

We would also like to express our sincere appreciation to the team at The Guilford Press for their enthusiastic support of our vision, helping us turn it into reality. A special thanks is due to the incomparable Kitty Moore, whose humor kept us uplifted and motivated throughout this process.

On a personal note, I, Shireen, wish to thank my husband for his unwavering support and encouragement, as well as for being a true coparent through thick and thin. I also express my gratitude to my children for providing countless opportunities to practice these skills, and for being lovable goofballs. Finally, I extend my appreciation to Jesse for his inspiration and for making the trek to New Jersey for many work dates.

I, Jesse, would like to thank my family and friends for their consultation and emotional support throughout this process. I would also like to acknowledge the brilliant Gerhard Assini for his contributions to the artwork. Special thanks to Shireen, who not only made sure I was well fed during every New Jersey work session, but also changed the trajectory of my life by introducing me to the fundamentals of cognitive-behavioral therapy and teaching me nearly everything I know about DBT.

INTRODUCTION

Hello! You picked up this book for a reason. Our guess is that you're struggling in some way. Perhaps you're agonizing over a tumultuous relationship, or maybe you feel lonely and sad that you're not in a relationship. Perhaps you're losing sleep every night imagining all the things that could go wrong at work, or maybe you feel lost because you don't even know what type of work you'd enjoy. Maybe you're suffering with a chronic illness or chronic pain.

Maybe your struggle is more existential—you're overwhelmed by threats of climate crises, wars, infectious diseases, and political strife.

Or maybe it's a bit of all the above.

All of this feels awful. And yet . . . there's good news. The first bit of good news is that *you are not alone*. Everyone struggles in day-to-day life. When you're in the depths of despair, you might not always believe this, but trust us—it's a universal fact. We, the authors, struggle. Your neighbor struggles. The seemingly highly competent public figure struggles. The person who cut you off in traffic struggles. The struggle is real! Life is hard! When we're in pain it's easy to feel alone. So, if you decide to stop reading here and move on to another book, at least take away this fact: Everyone struggles in day-to-day life.

> *You are not alone. Everyone struggles in day-to-day life.*

Knowing that everyone is in this struggle together may help you feel less alone and less likely to think there is something wrong with you. That knowledge alone may lead to a greater sense of peace. Yet, the knowledge that everyone experiences problems does not actually help you solve yours.

So now for a second bit of good news. Any problem you're experiencing right now has likely been experienced by millions of others. Why is this good news? Because pain and suffering are universal experiences, scientists have worked tirelessly to develop and study psychological tools to reduce distress and improve mental health.

We created this book to bring some of these psychological tools together and present them to you in an easy-to-understand and user-friendly way.

These tools are skills from a psychological treatment called Dialectical Behavior Therapy (DBT). They have been studied extensively and shown to be helpful at reducing suffering for lots and lots of people, across many, many studies.

If you want to jump straight to those tools, you can! Feel free to head to the Pathways through Problems section or to the section called The Skills. If your need is a bit less urgent and you have a few moments, we'd like to share with you the basics and history of DBT. This information will provide a foundation for the rest of the book as well as a rationale for why we think these skills will help you in your everyday life.

The Basics of DBT

DBT was developed by the pioneering psychologist Dr. Marsha Linehan at the University of Washington in Seattle, beginning in the 1980s. Dr. Linehan initially developed DBT to treat suicidal women who met criteria for a diagnosis known as borderline personality disorder.

The first clinical trial of DBT was published in 1991. Since that time, many other studies have shown that DBT is an effective treatment for borderline personality disorder and for reducing suicidal behaviors. Individuals with borderline personality disorder now face a much more hopeful future than ever believed possible (provided they have access to quality DBT, of course).

You may be asking how this treatment, developed as a comprehensive therapy for such a severe and complex mental health problem, can be helpful for you in your everyday life. Fair question. DBT is based on two key assumptions that can be applied to all people, not just people with borderline personality disorder.

- Assumption 1. Most of our problems are a result of emotion dysregulation. That is, when we feel out of control with our emotions, we are more likely to engage in thoughts and behaviors that cause problems for us. We might drink too much, eat too much, text someone too much, lash out at someone, impulsively do something that isn't great for us, stay in bed all day because we feel depressed, or ruminate endlessly about everything that is wrong with our life. The list goes on.

- Assumption 2. These problems with emotion dysregulation happen because we lack skills to help us manage our emotions more effectively. In other words, we struggle and experience extreme distress because we don't know *how* to *do* other, more helpful behaviors. There are lots of reasons for this. Maybe we were never taught these skills by our parents, caregivers, or teachers. Maybe we had models of problematic behaviors from the adults in our lives (probably because they too never learned effective ways of coping!). Or maybe skillful behavior was just not emphasized or rewarded as we grew up.

Everyone—you, the authors, your friends, celebrities, everyone you meet—has skills deficits, regardless of the reason. By skills deficits, we mean not knowing how to do things differently. We want to emphasize how important it is to understand our problems as a result of skills deficits.

If you think the reason that you yell at your partner is because you're fundamentally a bad person, or the reason you're lonely is because "you're unlovable," or the reason you avoid exercise is because "you're just lazy," then you're likely to feel hopeless and give up on any possibility of change.

On the other hand, if we understand our problems as a result of skills deficits, we can then approach our behavior less judgmentally and with a more problem-solving attitude. We can become curious about our struggles instead of seeing them as just another reminder of our "badness."

As an example, think about moving to a small, foreign country whose language is spoken by only its people. You don't know a single word. We might say you have a skills deficit related to not knowing this foreign language. What's the best way to approach the situation? It would not be helpful or reasonable to berate yourself for never learning the language as a child. Instead, you would learn the language, one word at a time, starting with the words or phrases that will provide you the most help in as many situations as possible. In that sense, you slowly build up the skill of the language

> *If our problems are a result of skills we never learned, we can approach our behavior with a problem-solving attitude.*

with knowledge and practice. In this book, we are going to teach you the "language" of effective coping, one skill at a time.

These two, key DBT assumptions—that emotional problems are at the core of our suffering and that these problems are a result of not knowing what to do with them—led Dr. Linehan to develop dozens of evidence-based skills that comprise a major part of the treatment. In the standard form of DBT, people attend weekly skills-training sessions where they learn new skills each week. They are assigned homework to practice these skills during the week. There have been dozens of studies conducted on whether DBT skills work for a wide variety of problems. Overall, the research suggests that DBT skills are helpful for lots of different people with many different types of problems. For example, studies have shown that DBT skills are effective at reducing depression, anxiety, and impulsive behaviors.

Outside of the research, we can speak from personal experience. I, Shireen, first learned these skills from Marsha Linehan herself when I was her graduate student at the University of Washington 25 years ago. I can confidently say that I use these DBT skills every day. They have helped me (years ago) to tolerate the distress of dating, and (more currently) to reduce my stress related to parenting, negotiate for pay raises and other desirable work goals, manage my reactions to health problems, and navigate the challenges of everyday life.

I, Jesse, had the benefit of learning these skills from Shireen while a graduate student in clinical psychology at Rutgers University several years ago. I can, with equal confidence, say that I use these skills daily. They've helped me get through writing this book (just kidding, Shireen!), reduce conflict with my family, identify work and relationship goals, and truly, and I know this may sound annoying, live a more contented life.

Because we have seen the transformative power of DBT skills in our own lives, our students' and colleagues' lives, the lives of the clients we treat, and across numerous studies, we wanted to write a book that would make these skills more accessible for everyone. Our goal is *not* to provide standard DBT nor to replace a therapist. You may find that you need more help applying these skills to your own specific problems or that you need more help than what these skills provide. In that case, it is important for you to seek out mental health

> *Our goal is to teach these skills to you in ways that help you put them into practice immediately.*

treatment. Our goal is, however, to introduce you to these skills and teach them to you in ways that help you immediately put them into practice and observe their effects.

What Is a Dialectical Approach Anyway, and Why Is It Important?

DBT skills are now taught and practiced in many different settings, including therapy offices, schools, prisons, and hospitals. Most mental health clinicians are aware of them. But if you ask people what it means for the treatment to be considered "dialectical," most folks will still not know how to explain it. From the standpoint of getting the most out of these skills in your everyday life, we think it's important to understand the basics of dialectics. So, here's our crash course.

When Dr. Linehan began working with individuals diagnosed with borderline personality disorder, she applied standard cognitive-behavioral therapy strategies. At the time, cognitive-behavioral strategies consisted of helping people learn to change their thoughts and behaviors in order to reduce emotional pain. The idea was that if you could change the way you think (your interpretations) and what you do with your actions, you could change how you feel. However, she quickly found that a lot of her clients responded very negatively to this approach. They described feeling invalidated, often stating something like, "If I could change this easily, I would! You don't realize how hard this is." Additionally, this change-focused approach was challenged by clients who experienced parts of their lives that were less responsive to their attempts at change: abusive parents, traumatic histories, systemic inequality.

After some time hearing this feedback, Dr. Linehan decided to try a new method. She dropped the laser-focused approach to change and pivoted to something vastly different. At the time, she was studying Zen Buddhism, meditating extensively, and learning more about the value of being fully awake to the present moment. It occurred to her that she could try applying these principles of acceptance from Zen Buddhism with her clients. She started telling clients that, rather than constantly trying to change something about themselves, they could instead practice accepting their lives and themselves exactly as they are in this moment, without judgment. While clients reported that they found this approach more validating of their experience, over time they reported new frustrations. In addition to this validation, they wanted practical tools to help them change in ways that would move them closer to their goals.

Dr. Linehan realized then that focusing on *both* change *and* acceptance was necessary. She arrived at the notion of dialectics to help provide balance and recognize these two simultaneous goals. The dialectical philosophy, or worldview, comprises several tenets. While we won't review all of them, here are a few highlights:

1. Two contradictory views can both be true. For example, you can accept your life exactly as it is while also wanting it to be different.
2. Everything in the universe is interrelated.
3. Tension and polarization are inevitable.
4. The only constant in life is change.

What does all this have to do with the skills you are about to learn and practice? Practicing these skills dialectically means practicing both acceptance skills and change skills and not being overly focused on either. Understanding and adopting a dialectical worldview also creates opportunities to think more dialectically—that is, to move from "black and white" thinking, which often creates misery and anger, and toward more balanced thinking. Finally, it means recognizing that a multitude of approaches are likely available to deal with any particular problem. Luckily for you, we provide these approaches for you here.

What Will I Be Learning?

The package of DBT skills covers four domains: mindfulness, interpersonal effectiveness, emotion regulation, and distress tolerance. We will be teaching you some of the DBT skills from each of these domains.* As a brief introduction, here's what each domain aims to teach.

* The full package of DBT skills with more than 225 handouts and worksheets describing how to use them can be found in Linehan's *DBT Skills Training Manual, Revised Edition,* and *DBT Skills Training Handouts and Worksheets, Revised Edition.*

- Mindfulness skills: Learn to be fully present in our daily lives, while letting go of judgments and distractions.
- Interpersonal effectiveness skills: Learn how to interact with others more effectively, specifically, how to ask for and say no to things in ways that increase the likelihood we'll get what we want.
- Emotion regulation skills: Learn to identify emotions that we're experiencing, change unwanted emotional experiences, and reduce our vulnerability to intense emotions.
- Distress tolerance skills: Learn to cope with difficult and distressing moments without doing anything to make the situation worse and learn to accept reality exactly as it is.

Let's circle back to the assumptions of DBT: The problems we experience are a result of emotion dysregulation that we don't know how to manage. Then it follows that learning more effective ways of coping will lead to fewer problems and greater likelihood of reaching our goals. You will find that you are capable of managing your feelings and behaviors. This in turn will also lead to greater sense of confidence and self-worth—what psychologists refer to as "self-efficacy."

How to Use This Book

We have structured this book as follows to aid in your learning and practice.

- Pathways through Problems: The first section guides you to particular skills to practice based on the unique circumstances of your problem. If you are new to DBT skills, these pathways will help you more readily identify the appropriate skill to use.
- The Skills: The second section provides a lesson on each of the 26 skills we cover in this book. For each skill, we describe why you might use it, what it is, when to use it (and when *not* to use it), how to know when it's working, what skills to use as alternatives, and illustrations that help show you how to practice. For some of the more complex skills, we have

also added illustrated "In Practice" pages to show an example of what the skills might look like when they're used successfully.

- The End Is Just the Beginning: The final section provides information on how to adopt these skills in ways that lead to a more balanced and effective life. In addition to using these skills in response to difficult moments, you can also use them in proactive ways, day to day. Through DBT skills, we hope to help you cultivate a feeling of self-efficacy in all moments of your life. You'll learn that, even when faced with problems, you can survive and handle them in ways that you can ultimately be proud of.

There is no magic potion or set of skills that will end all our struggles, distress, and pain and create a life of never-ending peace and contentment. Yet, in this book you will find the tools to cope with whatever your life throws at you. When asked to sign copies of her book, Marsha Linehan would write "wishing you skillful means." Thank you for picking up this book. We hope that *you* find skillful means to help you navigate life's challenges and discover a deeper sense of resilience and happiness.

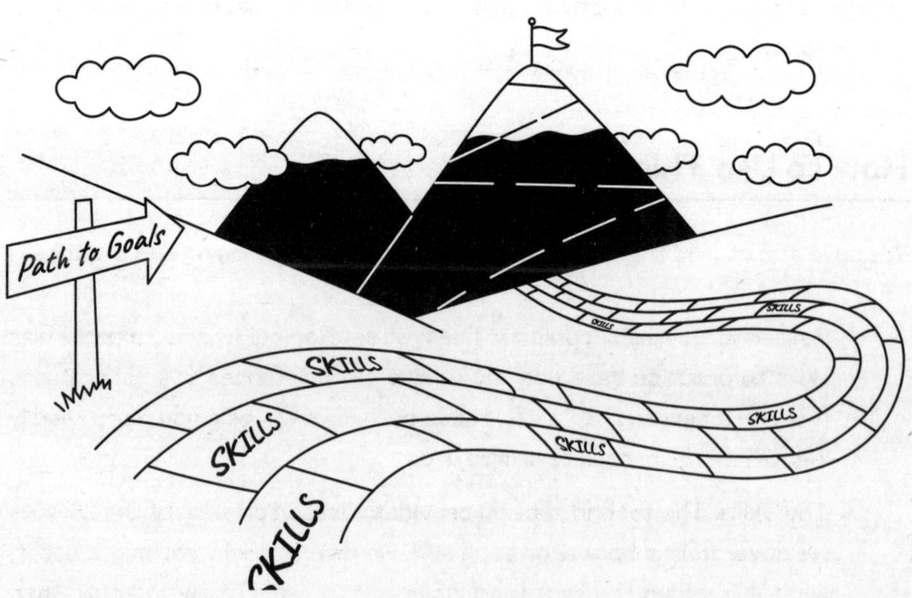

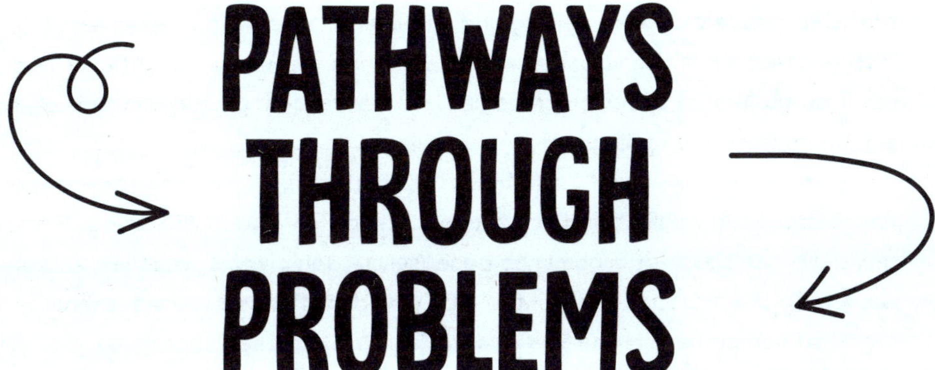

PATHWAYS THROUGH PROBLEMS

DBT has a lot of skills—each one valuable in its own way! But when you're in high distress or just starting out, figuring out which skill to use (and when) can feel overwhelming. So, we made it easier for you. We created four "pathways through problems" to help you get from problem to solution as quickly as possible. Follow the flowchart, answer key questions, and land on a skill to try.

The first pathway, "I'm in a crisis," is for moments when you're feeling overwhelmed or distressed by something happening right now. In these situations, you want to respond skillfully to distress, rather than engage in behaviors that could make things worse. By *crisis,* we mean any situation that feels deeply upsetting in the moment—perhaps you just got some terrible news, a relationship ended, you're struggling with a work or school assignment, or you're spiraling into existential dread. Whatever your crisis, use this path to find a skill and manage your distress in this particular moment.

The second pathway, "I'm ruminating," covers the all-too-common problem of getting stuck in repetitive, unhelpful thoughts. Maybe you've noticed replaying the same scenario over and over, feeling trapped in a mental loop that's getting you nowhere. Rumination can block effective action and pull you away from what's actually happening in the present moment. This path helps you determine if your thinking is leading to effective problem solving or if you need to throw yourself into another activity to break the cycle.

The third pathway, "I don't want to feel this emotion," is for those moments when you're experiencing an emotion that feels painful, uncomfortable, or just unwanted. This is a common experience! This path starts by helping you identify what you're currently feeling and whether that emotion makes sense (or "fits the facts") of the situation you're in. Once you know these two things, you'll be guided to specific strategies—either to change the emotion or to accept what you're feeling.

And the last pathway, "I'm fighting with someone," is for those times when you're caught in conflict and don't know how to manage it effectively. Sometimes we get stuck in arguments because we don't know what we actually want from the situation. This path helps you identify what you want from the start, so you can approach the situation with a strategy that gives you the best chance of managing it effectively.

These pathways are here to help you find the right skill for you in the moment. However, it's really important that you know that these paths are not meant to be prescriptive (as in "you must do this!"). There is no one-size-fits-all approach. If a path leads to a skill that wouldn't be effective right now, try something else.

As you work your way through the skills in this book, you'll start to develop your own pathways through problems. You'll figure out what works best for *you* in the different situations that *you're* in. If you ever get stuck, just come back to one of these pathways and see if any new options show up for you.

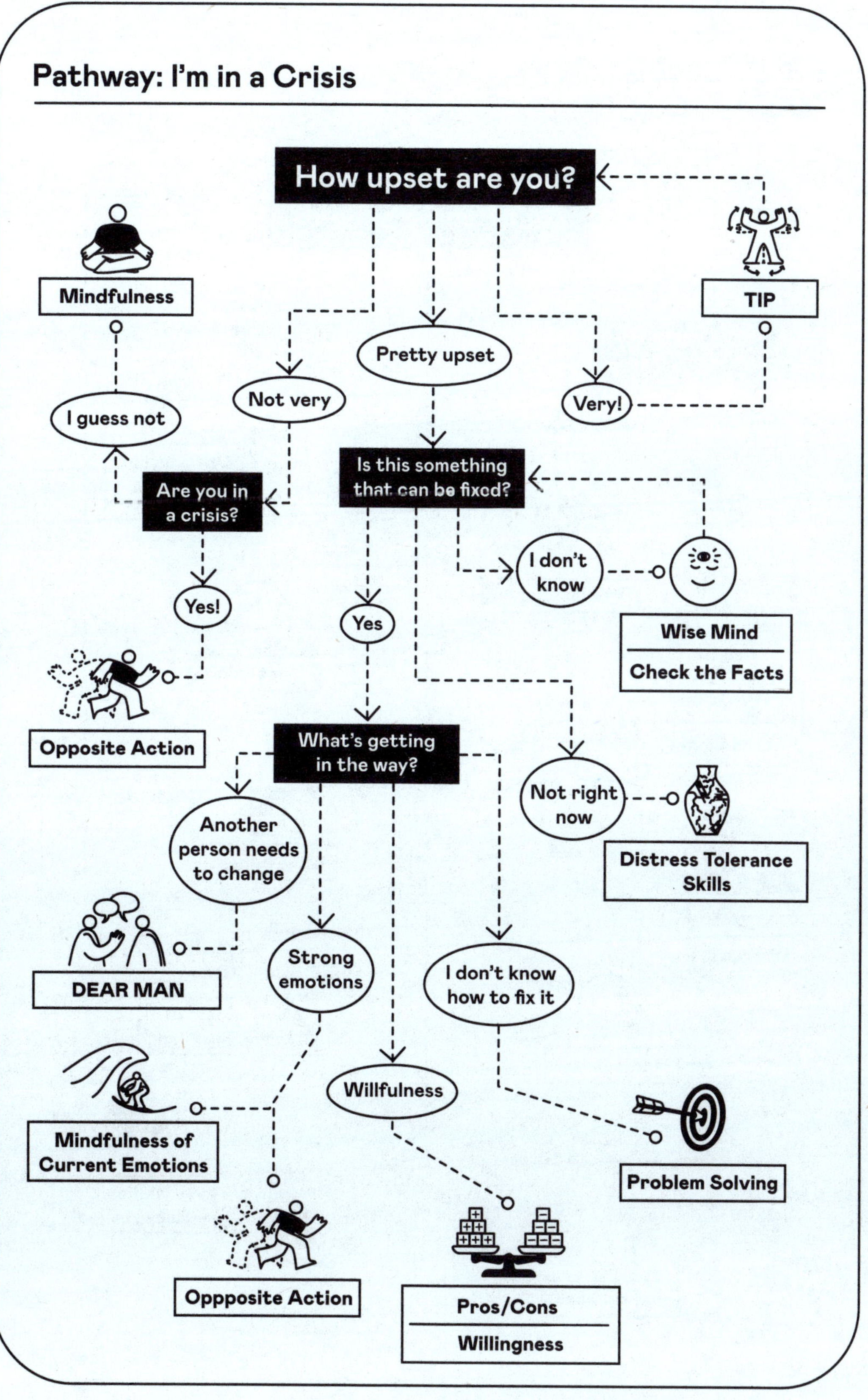
Pathway: I'm in a Crisis
How upset are you?
Mindfulness
TIP
Pretty upset
Not very
Very!
I guess not
Is this something that can be fixed?
Are you in a crisis?
I don't know
Yes!
Yes
Wise Mind
Check the Facts
Opposite Action
What's getting in the way?
Not right now
Another person needs to change
Distress Tolerance Skills
Strong emotions
I don't know how to fix it
DEAR MAN
Willfulness
Mindfulness of Current Emotions
Problem Solving
Oppposite Action
Pros/Cons
Willingness

Pathway: I'm Ruminating

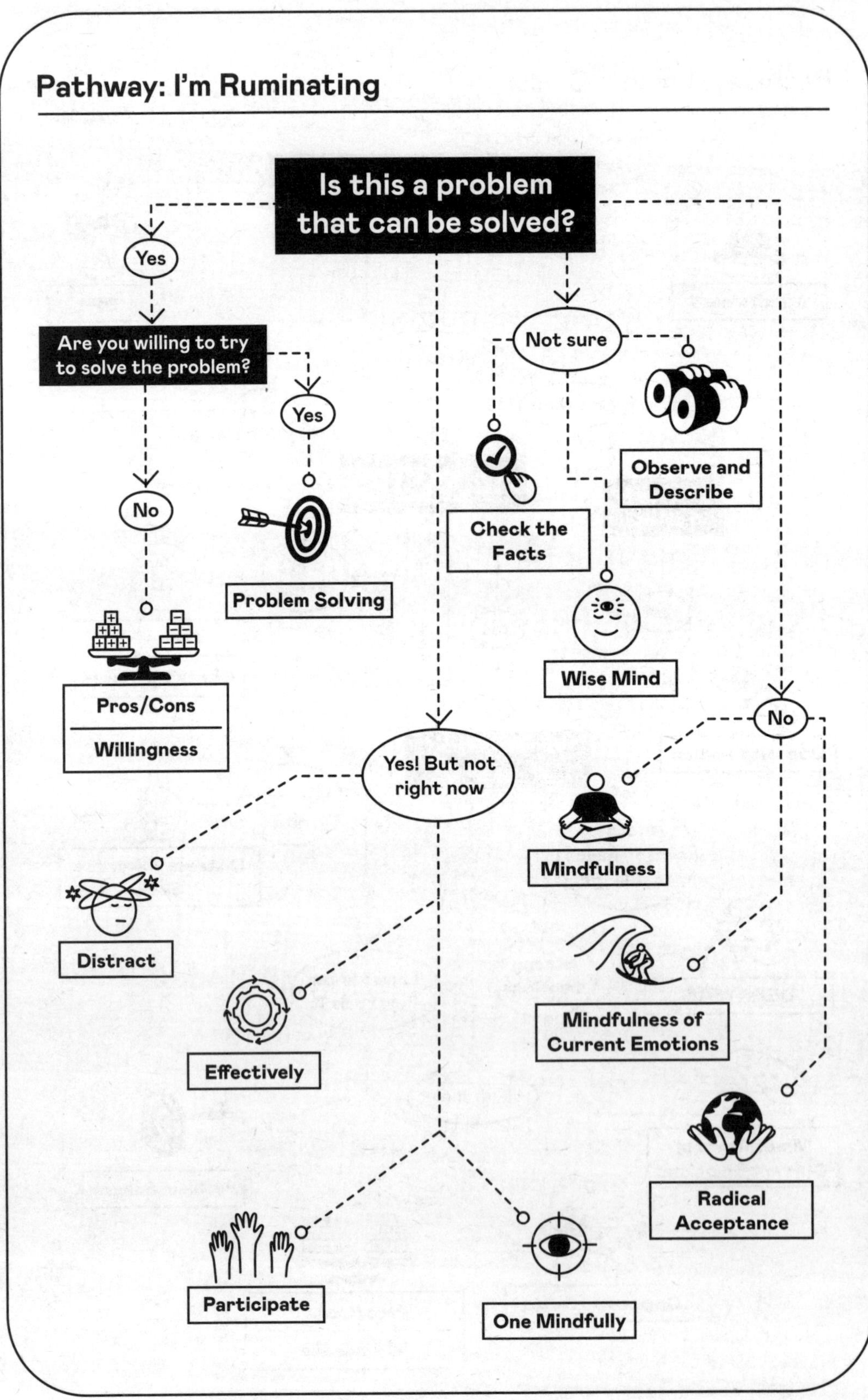

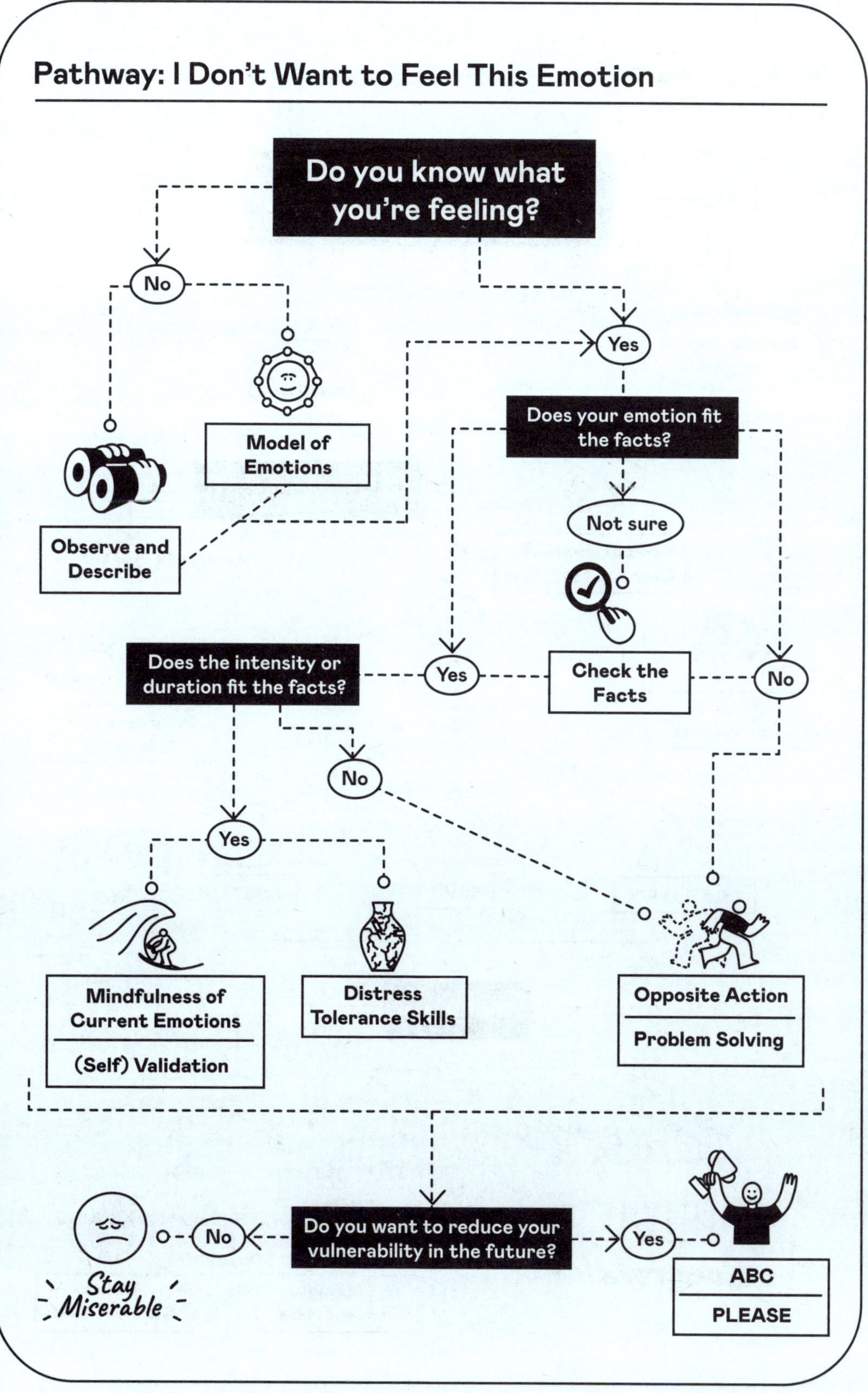
Pathway: I Don't Want to Feel This Emotion
Do you know what you're feeling?
No
Yes
Model of Emotions
Observe and Describe
Does your emotion fit the facts?
Not sure
Check the Facts
Yes
No
Does the intensity or duration fit the facts?
No
Yes
Mindfulness of Current Emotions
(Self) Validation
Distress Tolerance Skills
Opposite Action
Problem Solving
Do you want to reduce your vulnerability in the future?
No
Yes
Stay Miserable
ABC
PLEASE

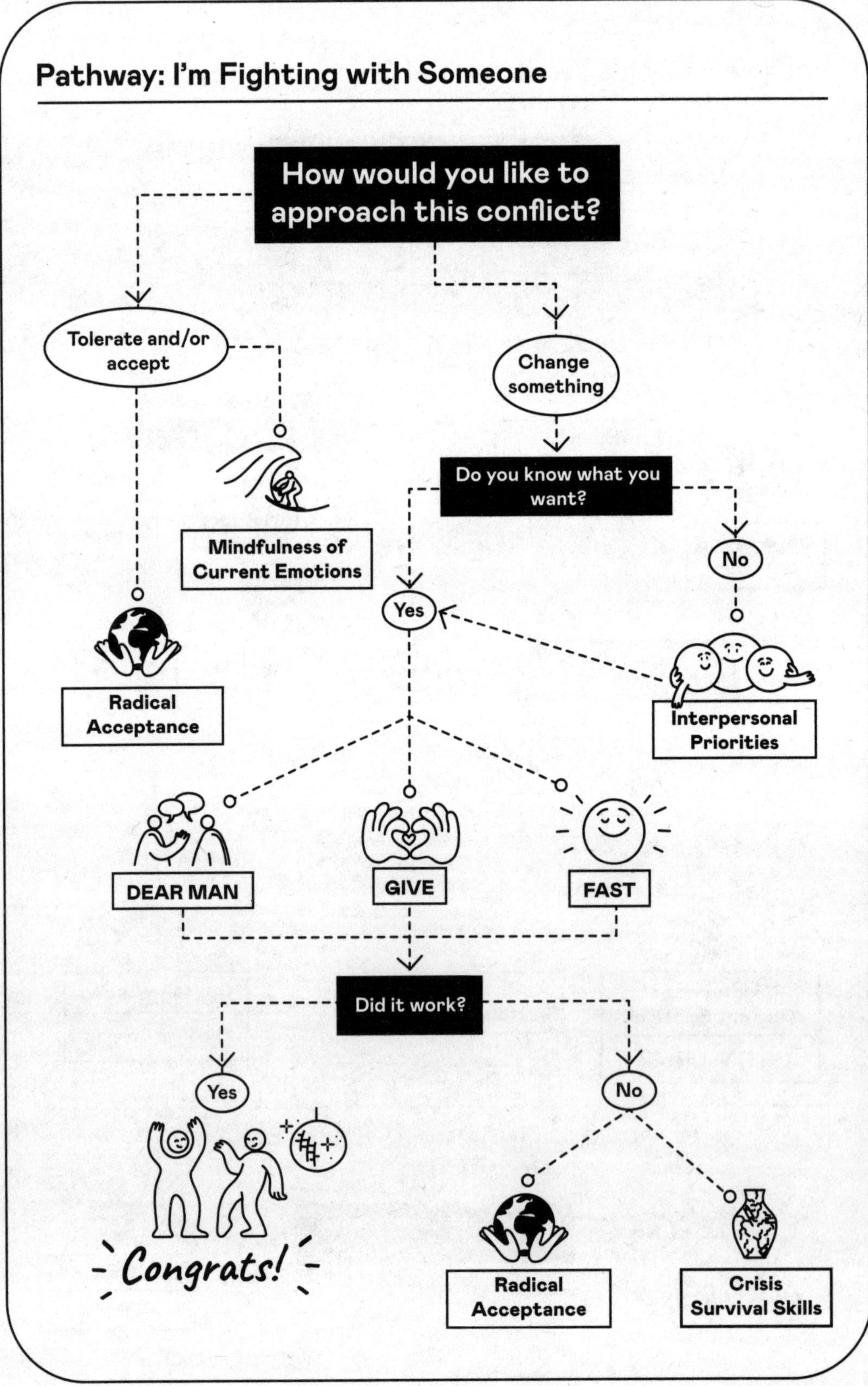
Pathway: I'm Fighting with Someone
How would you like to approach this conflict?
Tolerate and/or accept
Change something
Mindfulness of Current Emotions
Do you know what you want?
No
Yes
Radical Acceptance
Interpersonal Priorities
DEAR MAN
GIVE
FAST
Did it work?
Yes
No
Congrats!
Radical Acceptance
Crisis Survival Skills

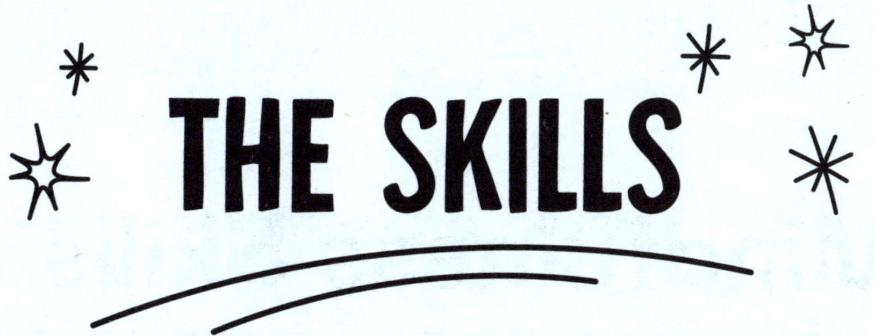

THE SKILLS

Mindfulness Skills

AN OVERVIEW

Mindfulness and meditation are pretty ubiquitous terms. Even if you do not practice yourself (yet), you have likely heard of meditation being taught in various contexts, such as in schools, companies, prisons, or with sports teams and high-level executives. Maybe you've seen (or use) one of the dozens of websites or apps that are designed to teach mindfulness and help people practice more consistently. Or you may know of mindfulness or meditation being taught in the context of religious practice. With all that, most people reading this book likely have some familiarity with principles of mindfulness.

That said, learning the specific DBT mindfulness skills can be helpful to all people, whether you are a complete newcomer to mindfulness or a seasoned meditator. In DBT, we teach mindfulness as opposed to more formal meditation practices. A standard definition of *mindfulness,* attributed to Dr. Jon Kabat-Zinn, is "awareness that arises through paying attention, on purpose, in the present moment, non-judgmentally." The DBT mindfulness skills provide concrete ways in which to practice achieving this awareness in daily living. None of them requires sitting on a meditation cushion for hours. All of them can be practiced in virtually any moment of the day.

There are seven mindfulness skills, or ways to practice. These seven skills are named Wise Mind, Observe, Describe, Participate, Nonjudgmentally, One-Mindfully, and Effectively. You can think of them in three groups.

- Wise Mind is a standalone skill that refers to feeling centered and wise in one's mind, body, and soul. Wise Mind is achieved by being awake to and aware of what *is* in any given moment.
- Observe, Describe, and Participate are "What" skills. They refer to *what* we do when we practice being mindful.
- Nonjudgmentally, One-Mindfully, and Effectively are "How" skills. They refer to *how* we practice mindfulness.

If that doesn't make sense now, don't worry. You'll see more as we describe these skills more fully and provide instructions for how to practice them.

Mindfulness skills are often considered "core" skills in DBT because most of the other skills require some aspect of mindfulness. The idea is that if we use these skills in our daily lives, we will cultivate a greater sense of awareness of this one moment. This awareness will allow us to respond to what is *actually happening* in this moment, as opposed to a fantasy of what we think is happening or what we wish would happen. This in turn will lead to a more centered and wise presence and ultimately reduce our experiences of struggle and distress.

WISE MIND

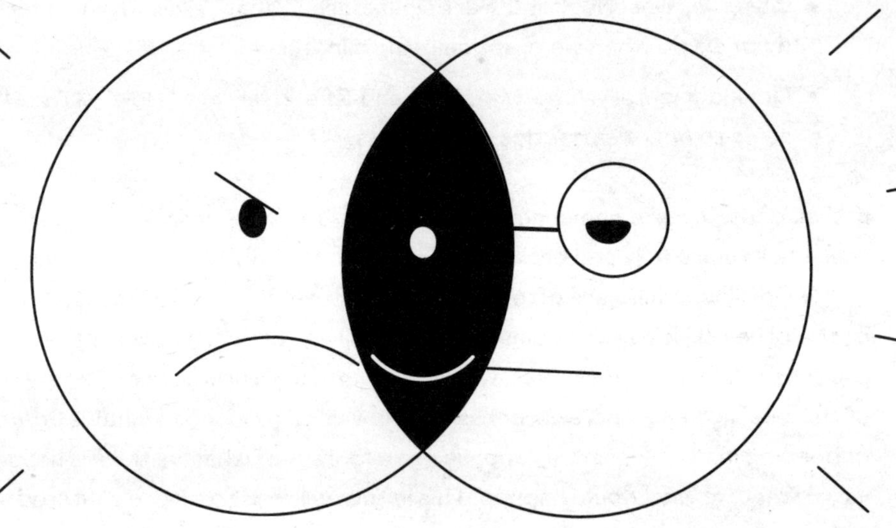

Why Use Wise Mind?

Wise Mind is good for when we want to get centered or wise. This is usually when we are facing an important decision, when we are trying to determine an effective course of action, or when we are stressed.

When to Use Wise Mind

☑ **Use when:**

- You are faced with a difficult decision and don't know what to do.
- You feel out of control with emotions.
- You feel out of control with reason. This is harder to detect, though a clue is when others tell us we are unfeeling or cold.

☒ **Do NOT use when:**

You are trying to convince yourself that something you want to do is Wise Mind. This is usually Emotion Mind masquerading as Wise Mind. For example, you might tell yourself that Wise Mind is saying you should stay with an abusive partner, when really fear is driving your decision. Instead, see what decision you come to when you practice Wise Mind.

WISE MIND refers to a state of mind, or state of being, where you feel the wisest and make the best (most effective) decisions. Wise Mind is often described as a centered, gut feeling experienced in the mind and body. Wise Mind involves integrating, or combining, two other states of mind that tend to take over when we're not effective: Emotion Mind and Reasonable Mind.

- Emotion Mind is the state of mind where your emotions control your thoughts, urges, and behaviors. When you're in Emotion Mind, your emotions dictate your responses, regardless of your long-term goals. For example, you might reach for a drink when stressed, even though you had previously committed to staying sober. Or you might stay in bed anxiously ruminating rather than getting up and exercising as you had planned. Or you might lash out in anger when someone criticizes you even though it strains the relationship.

- Reasonable Mind is the state of mind where reason and logic control your thoughts, urges, and behaviors. When you're in Reasonable Mind, facts and rationality dictate your responses, and emotions aren't really considered. For example, your friend calls you crying about a problem they're having and you disregard how they're feeling in order to get back to work. Or you calmly discuss breaking up with your partner without acknowledging the significant emotional impact.

Wise Mind represents the integration of Emotion Mind and Reasonable Mind. It is knowing the facts and logic in a situation, as well as tuning into emotional and sensory experiences, and using all that knowledge to make effective decisions. In Wise Mind, you might realize that anxious rumination is not helping you. With the clarity of Wise Mind, you get out of bed and put on your exercise clothes. Or you might say to yourself, *"My friend is important to me and is going through something hard. Let me put my work aside for a few minutes and attend to them fully so that I can be supportive. I'll return to my work when we're done."*

How to Know If Wise Mind Is Working

Often the experience of Wise Mind is associated with a feeling of calm and deep knowing. That feeling also lasts beyond the initial moment (to differentiate it from being an impulsive choice).

How to: Wise Mind

Identify the state of mind you're currently in.

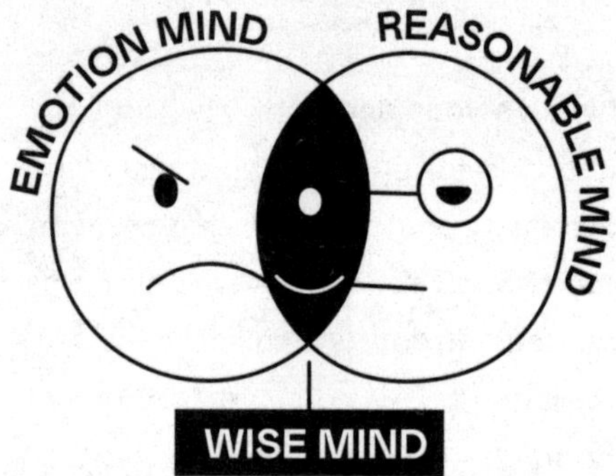

Are you feeling out of control with emotions? Are you having a hard time feeling anything?

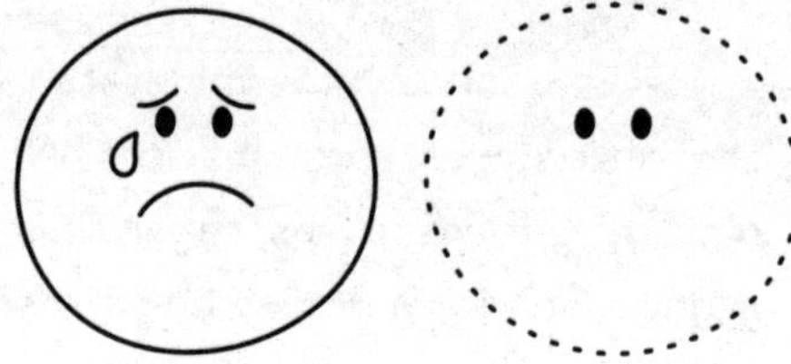

Sometimes just recognizing that we are NOT in **Wise Mind** can help us.

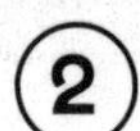

To access your **Wise Mind**, focus on the area in your body that you consider your "center."

This varies by person—your center could be in your abdomen, your heart, or your forehead (like the "third eye").

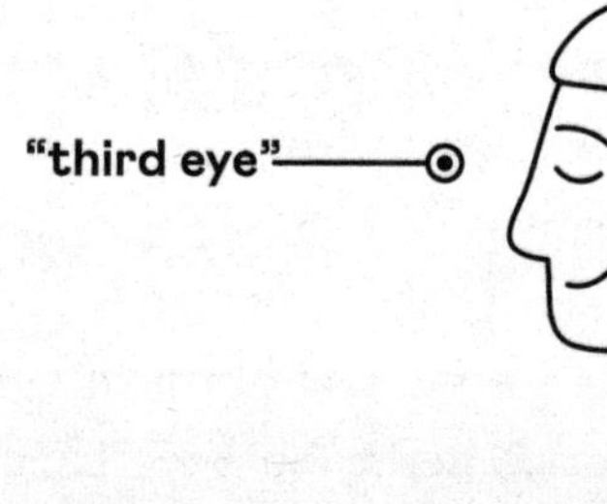

TRY THIS

Breathe into your center, noticing the sensations of your body. Does your breath slow down? Do you feel less tense and more relaxed?

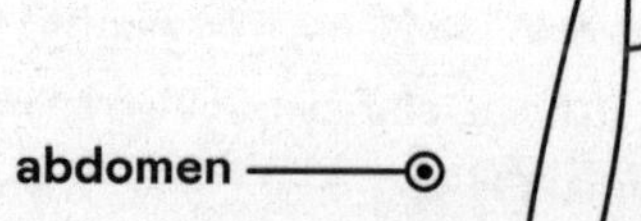

You can use visualization exercises like imagining yourself walking down a spiral staircase to your very center, becoming calmer and more settled as you go.

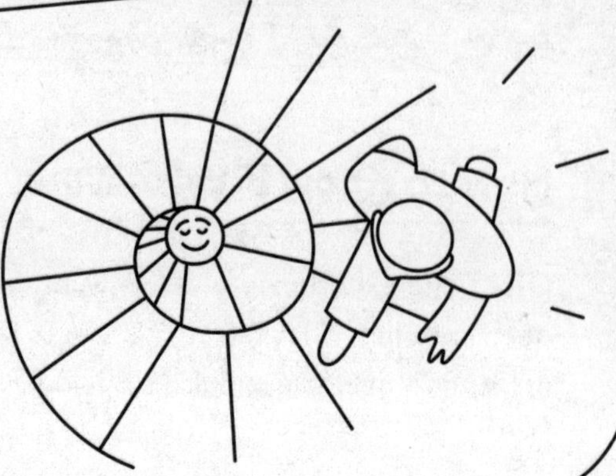

3 If you are facing a difficult decision, ask your **Wise Mind**.

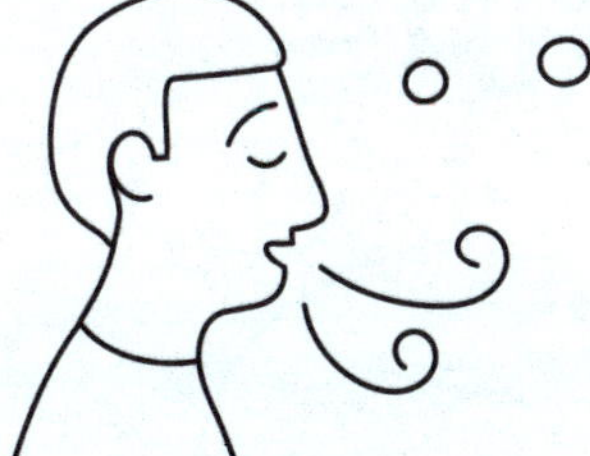

As you breathe in, ask yourself the question. As you breathe out, see what arises.

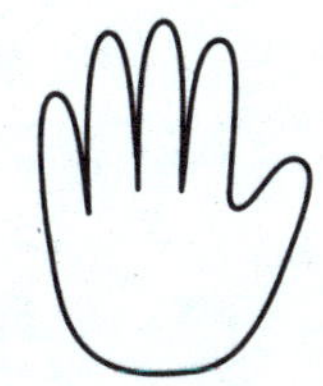

PAUSE
Do not force the answer. See what comes to you.

4 If you're feeling overwhelmed, numb, or disconnected, breathe into your center.

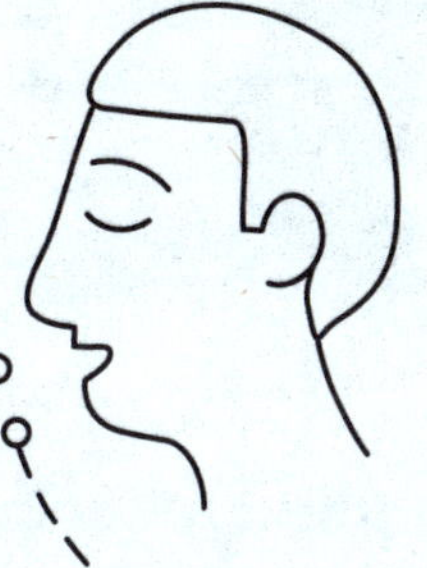

Silently say the word "Wise" on the inhale and exhale the word, "Mind."

5 Accessing **Wise Mind** can be difficult when we're:

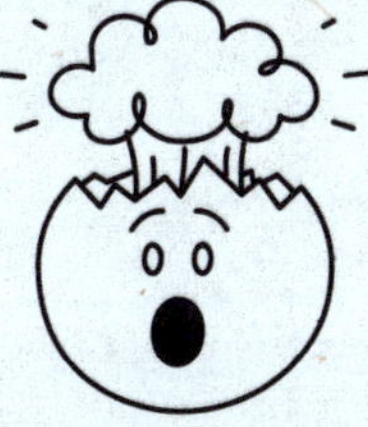
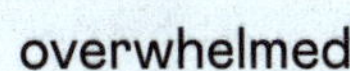

overwhelmed

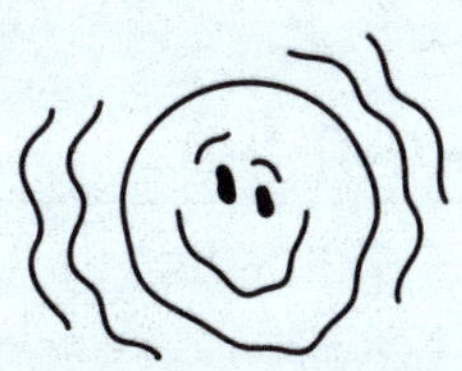

intoxicated

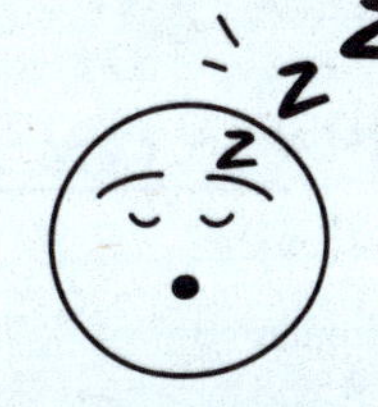

overtired

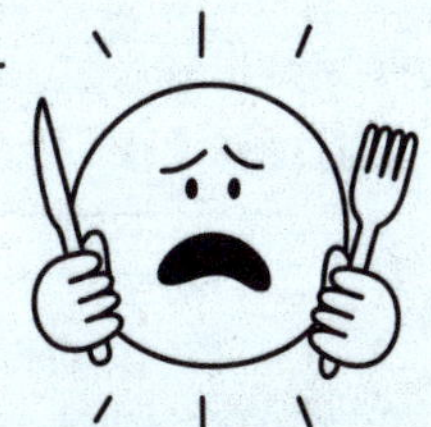

hungry

Consider addressing these factors first (like with the **PLEASE** skill, page 84) and then coming back to **Wise Mind** practice.

When Wise Mind isn't effective, practice these skills:
PLEASE · DISTRACT · TIP · PROS/CONS

OBSERVE AND DESCRIBE

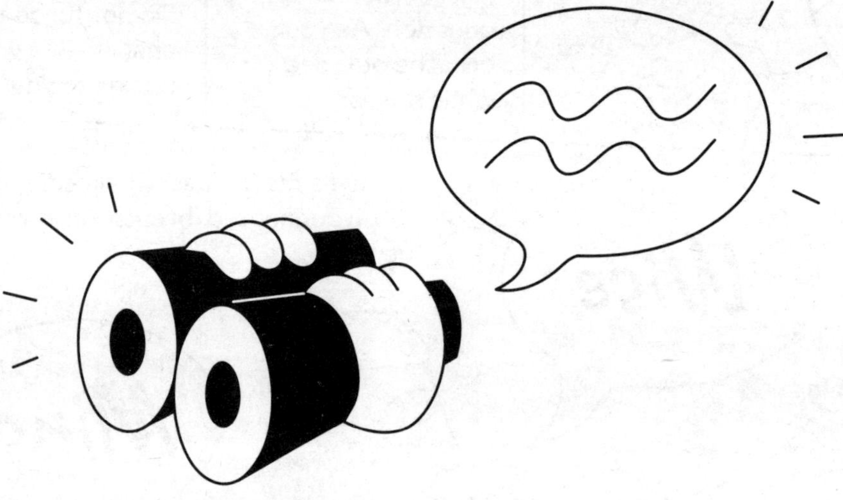

Why Use Observe and Describe?

Observe and Describe anchor us to the present moment, which is helpful when our brain is overtaken by thoughts about the past or future. They also allow us to gain some distance and perspective from what we are experiencing in the present moment.

When to Use Observe and Describe

☑ **Use when:**

Anytime! Decades of research on mindfulness suggest that the more we practice these core skills, the more regulated and at ease we will feel. Practice Observe and Describe in moments of distress so that you can notice and label what is truly happening (the "facts") versus the fictions or stories that exist in your head.

☒ **Do NOT use when:**

It is more effective to act than to step back and observe. If a fire breaks out near you, it is not the time to Observe and Describe—it's the time to put out the fire or get away!

OBSERVE AND DESCRIBE are critical mindfulness skills. In DBT, they are labeled mindfulness "What" skills because they are *what* you do when you practice.

Observe involves determining an object of focus and just noticing it, at the level of sensation. Sometimes this is referred to as "wordless watching." The object of focus could be your breath, sounds, what you're looking at, something that you are eating or drinking, your body sensations, or even things that you smell. The quality of noticing is just allowing whatever shows up to show up, without holding onto or pushing away any thought or sensation.

Describe is the practice of adding words to your Observe experience. So when mindfully walking outside, Describe might be:

"Blue bird flying overhead"

"Smell of freshly mowed grass"

"Cool breeze against my skin"

"Sound of tires on roads"

Describe is adding "just the facts" to our experience, and not adding interpretations or judgments. We say "blue bird flying overhead" and not "beautiful bird" or "annoying loud bird." We can instead describe our interpretations or judgments as thoughts; for example, "I'm noticing the thought 'the bird is too loud' went through my mind."

Observe and Describe can be used with emotional experiences. For instance, rather than being consumed by sadness, Observe and Describe what sadness feels like in the body. We can label "heaviness in chest," "slow movement," "thoughts of worthlessness," "urges to get back in bed."

How to Know If Observe and Describe Are Working

The experience of redirecting our attention to this one moment (or this one object of focus) *is* the practice. It is not about getting rid of all distractions, but rather about noticing the distractions as they occur and returning to your focus. Instead of using "feeling better" as your goal, the skills of Observe and Describe are "working" if you notice your experience exactly as it is, without adding on.

How to: Observe and Describe

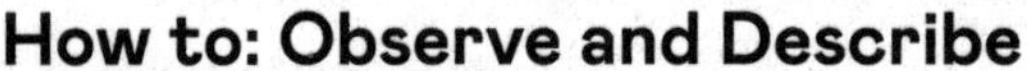

1. To practice **Observe**, notice your sensations. Pick a sensation or an object on which to focus and just notice.

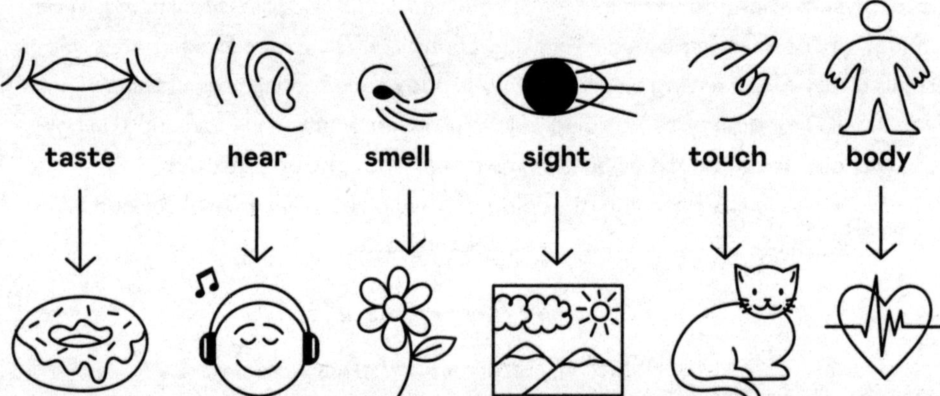

TRY THIS
Allow sensations, thoughts, and images to flow through you.

2. Pay attention to whatever arises in this one moment.

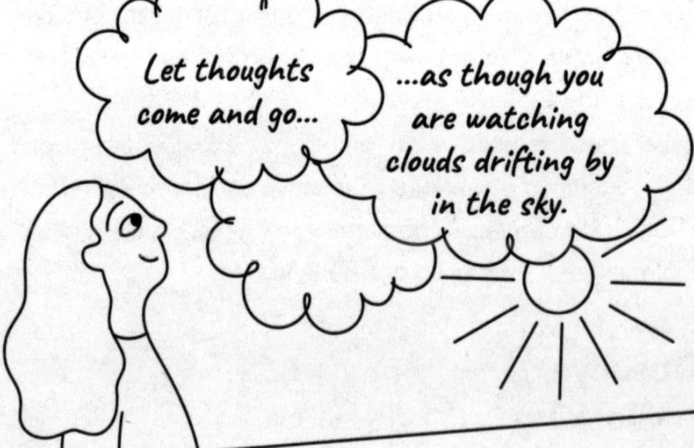

PAUSE

Avoid holding onto any single sensation or thought.

3. When you get distracted, just notice that and gently bring your attention back to the present and your sensations.

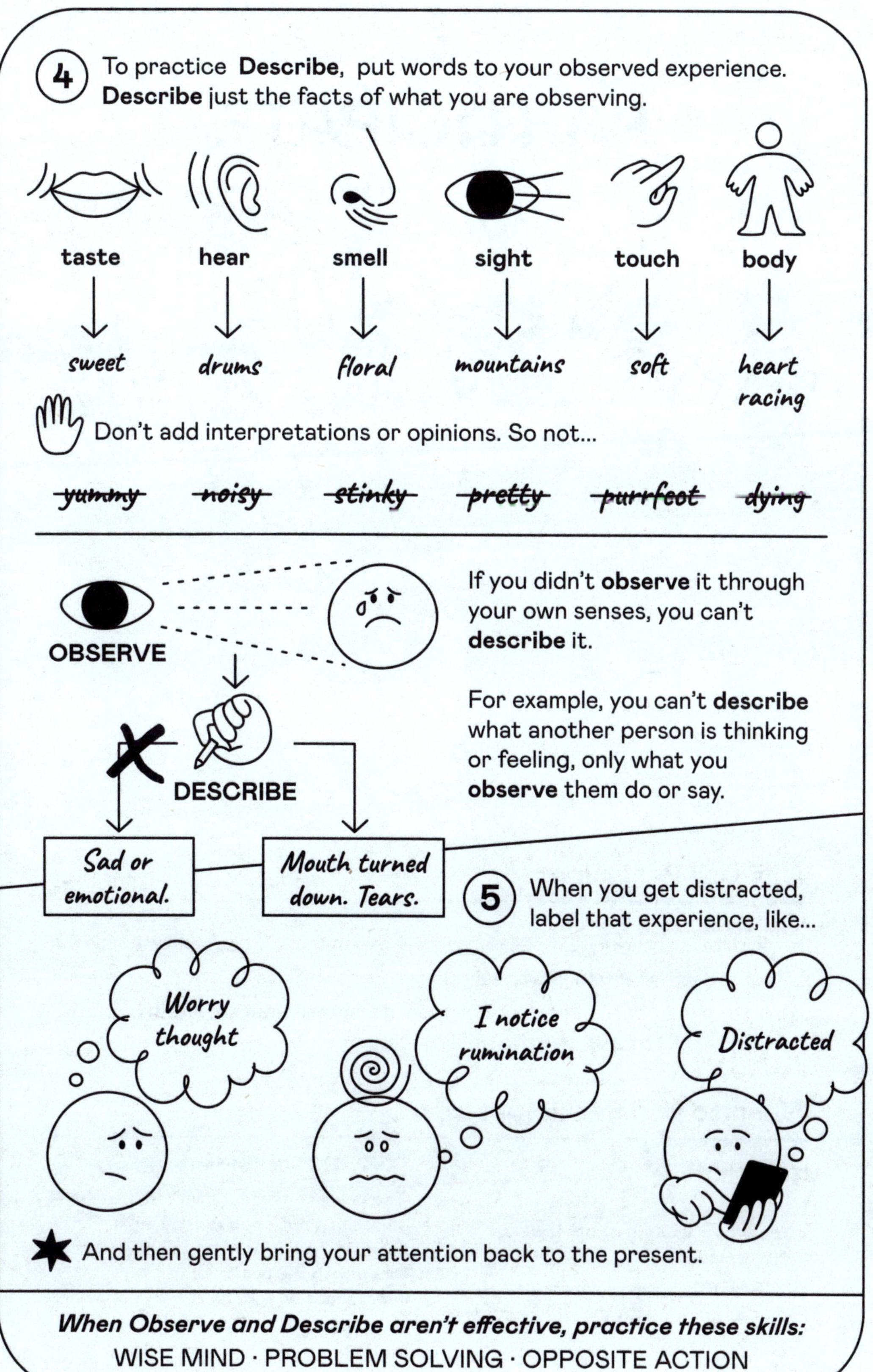
4
To practice Describe, put words to your observed experience.
Describe just the facts of what you are observing.
taste
hear
smell
sight
touch
body
sweet
drums
floral
mountains
soft
heart racing
Don't add interpretations or opinions. So not...
yummy
noisy
stinky
pretty
purrfect
dying
OBSERVE
DESCRIBE
Sad or emotional.
Mouth turned down. Tears.
If you didn't observe it through your own senses, you can't describe it.
For example, you can't describe what another person is thinking or feeling, only what you observe them do or say.
5
When you get distracted, label that experience, like...
Worry thought
I notice rumination
Distracted
And then gently bring your attention back to the present.
When Observe and Describe aren't effective, practice these skills:
WISE MIND · PROBLEM SOLVING · OPPOSITE ACTION

PARTICIPATE

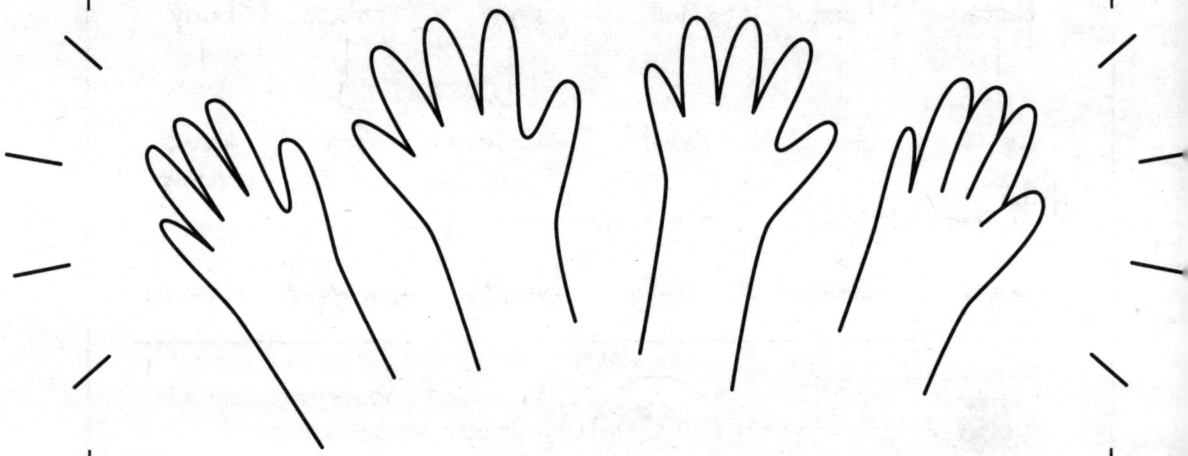

Why Use Participate?

Participate is entering completely into the experience of the moment with full awareness and intention. If we truly throw ourselves into this one moment, we can often find a sense of pleasure or ease, no matter what we are doing.

When to Use Participate

☑ **Use when:**

- Anytime!
- You are ruminating or otherwise distressed.
- You want to increase your sense of pleasure or joy with the moment.

☒ **Do NOT use when:**

The present moment involves something not good for you. For example, do not use Participate when faced with the option to use harmful substances or engage in risky behavior.

PARTICIPATE is another mindfulness "What" skill and is the act of throwing yourself 100% into whatever you're doing in this moment and being one with the flow. It is sometimes considered the ultimate form of mindfulness because it's applying "be in this moment" to any activity. Most of the time we are not actually in the moment. We are thinking about other things, planning the next thing, or wishing we were doing something else. Even when the current moment is pleasurable, we often struggle to stay fully present. We get distracted by other thoughts or we worry about when the moment will end.

For example, to practice Participate in a conversation with someone, you might put away all distractions, like phones, and just be with the other person and the conversation. It would mean being fully present without planning what you're going to say next or worrying about something that happened earlier. Participate involves riding out urges to do anything else and refocusing on this one moment again and again.

Using the skill of Participate, we engage fully with this one moment whether it is something we like (laughing with friends), something we don't like (vacuuming), or something we feel neutral about (walking from point A to point B). Participate is the opposite of multitasking. While many of us have been led to believe that multitasking is desirable, it turns out that multitasking is not so effective! We are all much more successful in our lives when we practice Participate.

Participate is bringing awareness to all aspects of our lives with intention. With practice, we become more present in our lives, open up opportunities for fun and enjoyment, and reduce our stress.

How to Know If Participate Is Working

Like the other core mindfulness skills, Participate "works" when you return over and over again to this one moment. If you continuously throw yourself into the moment, the skill is working to keep you centered in the here and now. The more you practice Participate, the faster you will notice when you're not in the present moment, and the easier it will become to bring your attention back to the present.

How to: Participate

1. Imagine what it would look like for you to be in this one moment, no matter what you're doing:

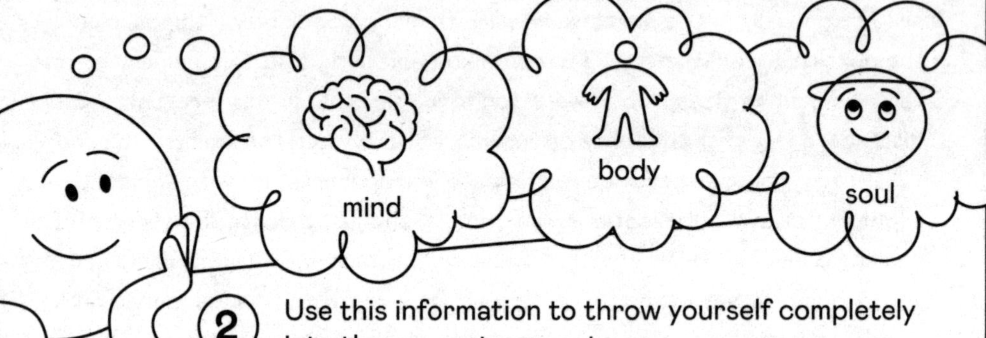

2. Use this information to throw yourself completely into the present moment.

NOT PARTICIPATE	PARTICIPATE
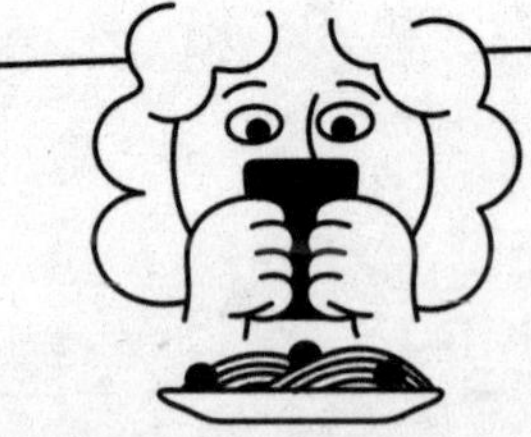 Sit alone at a party, worrying.	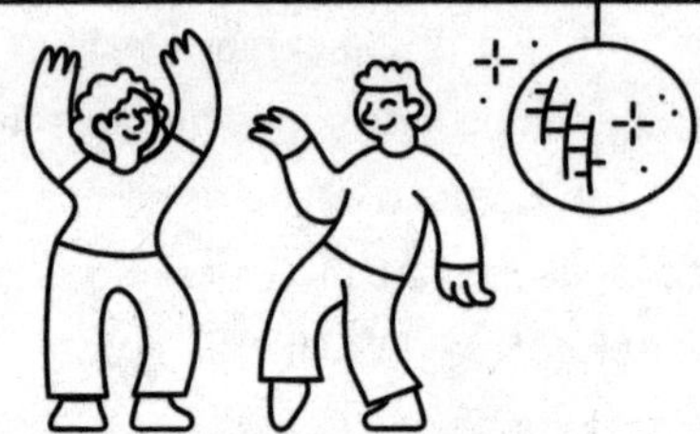 Dance with friends, letting go of self-consciousness.
Scroll through social media at dinner with family.	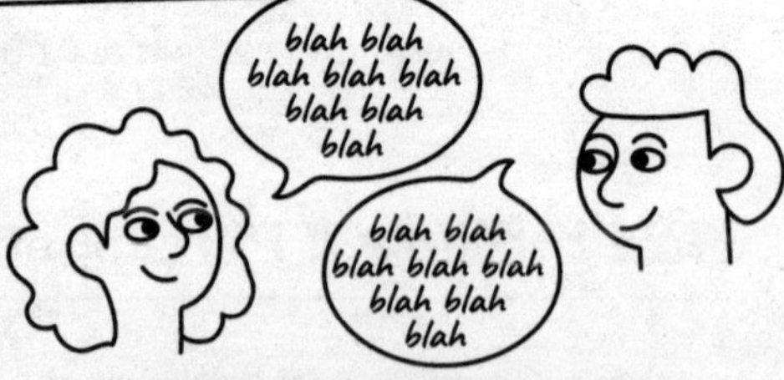 Engage fully in conversation with family.
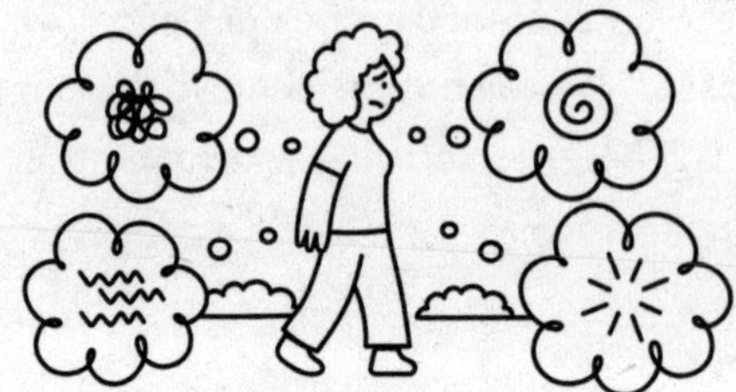 Ruminate while walking outside.	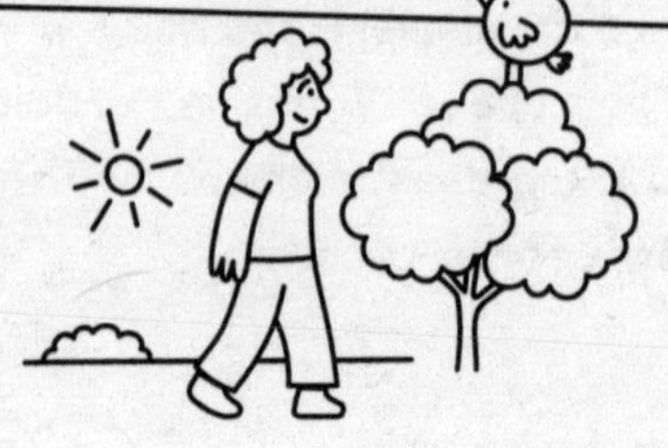 Take in all the sensory experiences while walking.

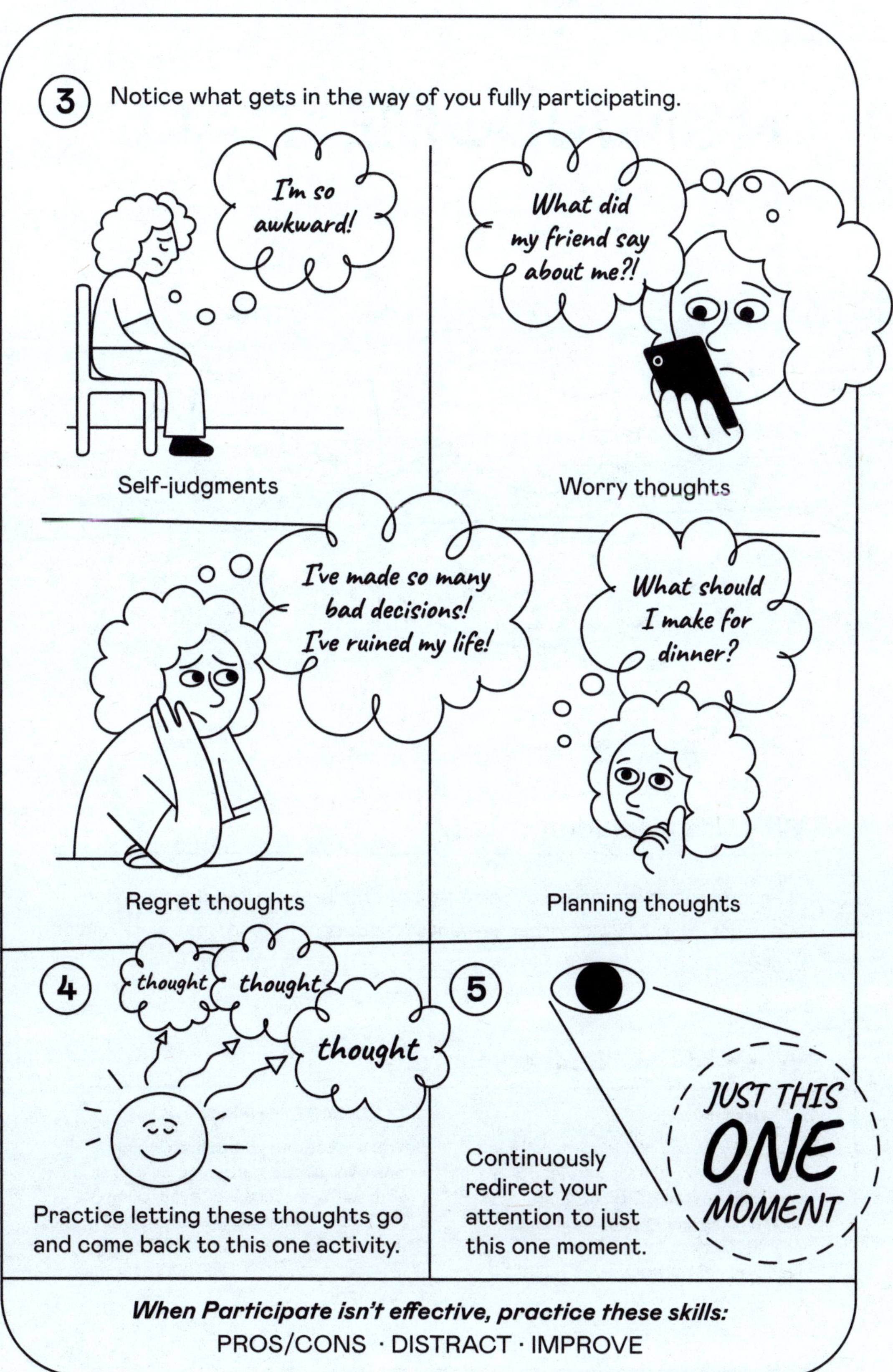
3
Notice what gets in the way of you fully participating.
I'm so awkward!
Self-judgments
What did my friend say about me?!
Worry thoughts
I've made so many bad decisions! I've ruined my life!
Regret thoughts
What should I make for dinner?
Planning thoughts
4
thought
thought
thought
Practice letting these thoughts go and come back to this one activity.
5
JUST THIS ONE MOMENT
Continuously redirect your attention to just this one moment.
When Participate isn't effective, practice these skills:
PROS/CONS · DISTRACT · IMPROVE

NONJUDGMENTALLY

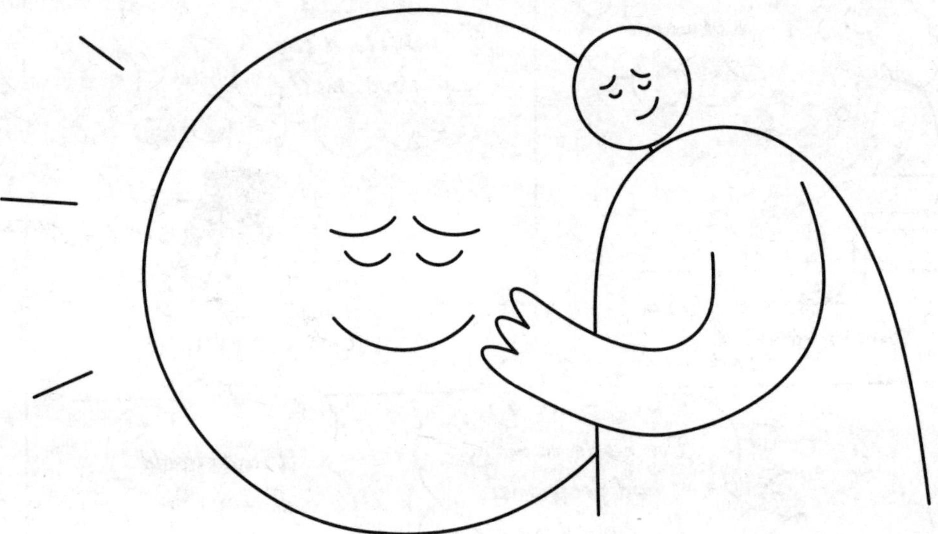

Why Use Nonjudgmentally?

Nonjudgmentally is good for seeing reality as it is and often aids in reducing our anger, irritability, or other unwanted emotions. It improves relationships too!

When to Use Nonjudgmentally

☑ **Use when:**

You find yourself making judgments about yourself, others, or life. So basically, anytime. Often, when you're experiencing anger, shame, or irritability, it's a cue that Nonjudgmentally can be of benefit.

☒ **Do NOT use when:**

You are forcing yourself to "think positive" about something or to get yourself from thinking "everything is awful" to "everything is wonderful." Instead, use it to get from "everything is awful" to "I don't like this experience right now."

NONJUDGMENTALLY is considered a mindfulness "How" skill: It's *how* we practice the other mindfulness skills. It may also be used outside the context of mindfulness activities. Nonjudgmentally refers to thinking about the world, ourselves, and others in a nonjudgmental manner without adding our opinions and interpretations. This is really hard! We often place values of "good" and "bad" on people, events, and things in subtle and not-so-subtle ways.

The skill of Nonjudgmentally is instead describing "just the facts." Aspiring to practice Nonjudgmentally in our lives can be a major game changer—we start to see how prevalent judgments are and how often those judgments are associated with emotions that cause distress, such as anger, envy, and sadness. By restating those judgments as nonjudgmental descriptions, we can gain a more accurate understanding of situations. While this doesn't make everything rainbows and unicorns, it will increase our capacity for empathy for ourselves and others.

Practicing Nonjudgmentally doesn't mean erasing our preferences. Instead, we preserve our preferences and state them nonjudgmentally. For example, "people who vote differently than me are such jerks" can be stated nonjudgmentally as "I wish everyone felt the same way as me about this issue" or "When people vote differently than me, I feel frustration and despair." Our likes and dislikes help inform important decisions and actions, so we don't want to get rid of them. Nonjudgmentally is not about getting rid of our likes or turning negatives into positives. It's about seeing the situation as it is, without adding layers of interpretation.

How to Know If Nonjudgmentally Is Working

On some occasions, a shift to thinking about things in a nonjudgmental way can lead to a huge sense of relief or a new perspective. When practiced regularly, Nonjudgmentally may also help gradually reduce the intensity of unwanted emotions and reduce tension in the body. However, practicing to be nonjudgmental is considered a lifelong skill. You don't just master it one day—you must continually work at it.

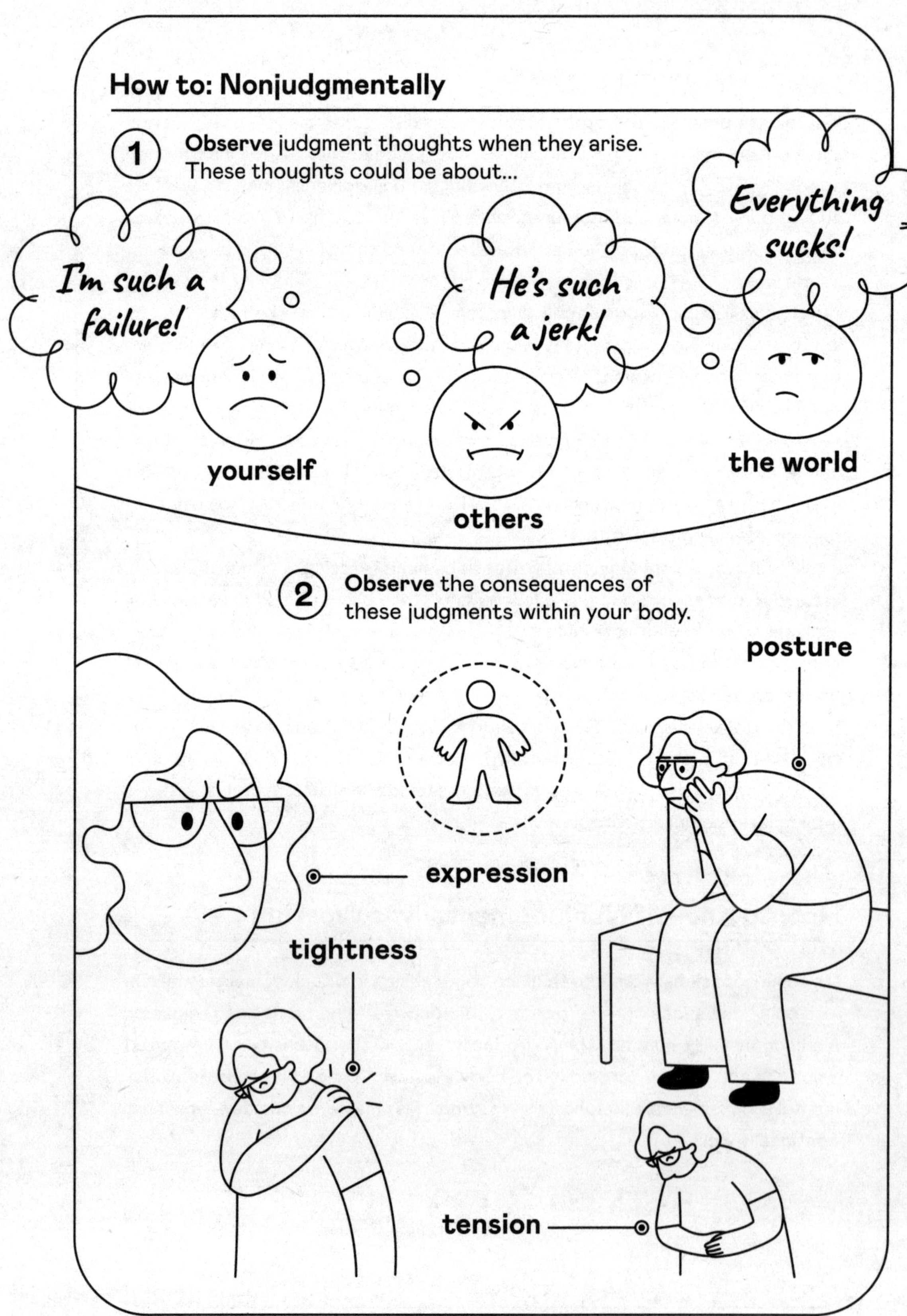
How to: Nonjudgmentally
1 Observe judgment thoughts when they arise.
These thoughts could be about...
I'm such a failure!
He's such a jerk!
Everything sucks!
yourself
others
the world
2 Observe the consequences of these judgments within your body.
posture
expression
tightness
tension

3 Use **Describe** and rephrase the judgmental thought into a nonjudgmental alternative.

judgment thought		nonjudgmental thought
I'm such a failure!	→	*I made an error and I feel disappointed.*
He's such a jerk!	→	*He interrupted me while I was talking, and I feel frustrated.*
Everything sucks!	→	*Things did not go as I had planned, and I feel stressed.*

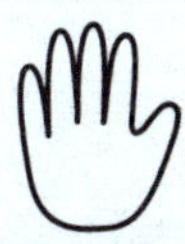

pause

Nonjudgmentally is not about turning a negative into a positive. We want to see the situation clearly without the added weight of judgmental labels.

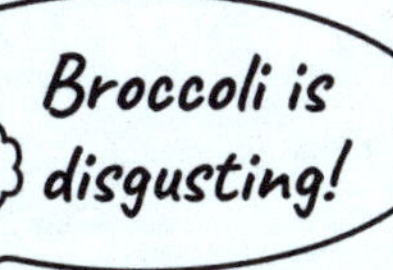

4 Most of us live in a sea of judgments. Practicing **Nonjudgmentally** can be like swimming against the tide.

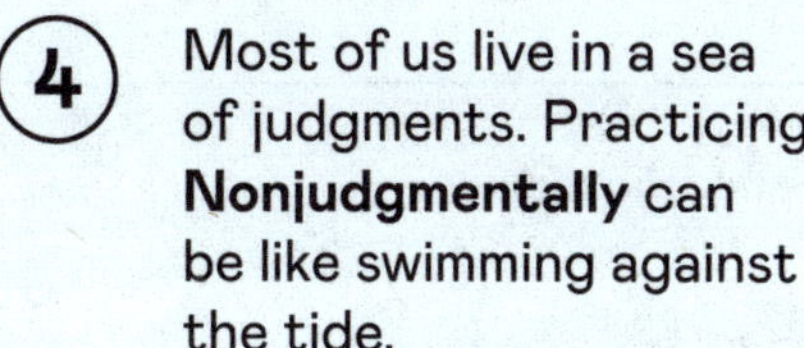

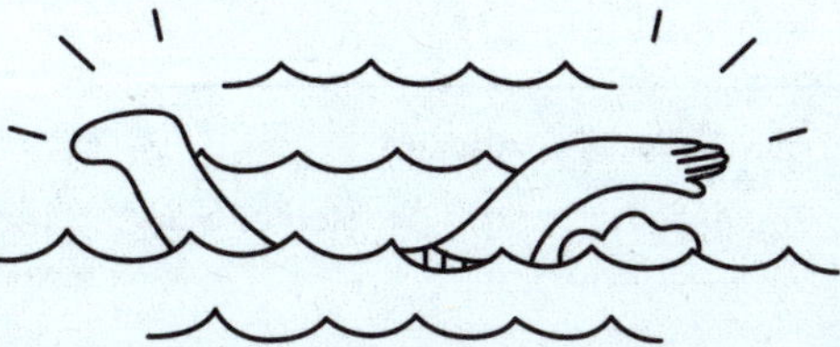

The more you practice, the stronger you'll become at noticing and changing judgments.

When Nonjudgmentally isn't effective, practice these skills:

DISTRACT · IMPROVE · RADICAL ACCEPTANCE (OF JUDGMENTS!) · WILLINGNESS

ONE-MINDFULLY

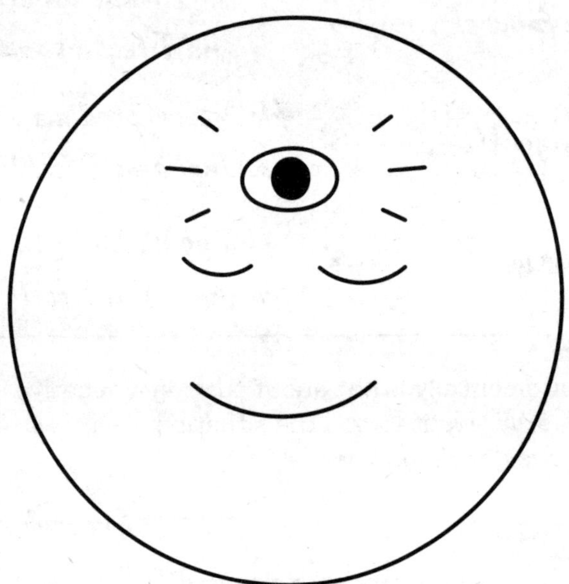

Why Use One-Mindfully?

One-Mindfully helps us get anchored to just this one moment.

When to Use One-Mindfully

☑ **Use when:**

Anytime! Especially useful when:

- You feel very scattered or easily distracted.
- Your thoughts and attention are being pulled into the past or the future.

☒ **Do NOT use when:**

You are engaging in problematic or risky behavior.

ONE-MINDFULLY is another mindfulness "How" skill, which means it's *how* you practice the other mindfulness skills. It refers to doing only one thing at a time with full attention.

One-Mindfully involves letting go of thoughts about the past and the future and, instead, refocusing our attention over and over to one activity. This skill takes effort. Distractions will inevitably arise, and when they do, you can gently observe them, let them go, and return your attention to the task at hand.

It's amazing how few things we are used to doing One-Mindfully, so practicing this skill might feel extremely difficult at first. We're often multitasking, and we have been (erroneously) taught that multitasking is productive and efficient. Instead, doing more than one thing at a time leads us to be more likely to make mistakes or to be forgetful and inattentive, thus leading us to be *less* effective. For example, have you ever noticed yourself trying to send a text and talk to a friend at the same time? And then you make an error in your text or miss something your friend said? Or both! Practicing One-Mindfully means *just* conversing with your friend or *just* texting, not trying to do both.

In addition to helping us be more effective, practicing One-Mindfully also tends to reduce stress or dissatisfaction. When we engage in whatever we're doing One-Mindfully, even if what we're doing is unpleasant or something we don't generally like, we can just notice what arises instead of adding thoughts of the future or past.

How to Know If One-Mindfully Is Working

Like all core mindfulness skills, One-Mindfully is working when we practice it! Just repeatedly bring your attention back to this one moment and this one activity.

How to: One-Mindfully

1. With intention, decide that you're going to practice **One-Mindfully**. You could practice **One-Mindfully** with any activity:

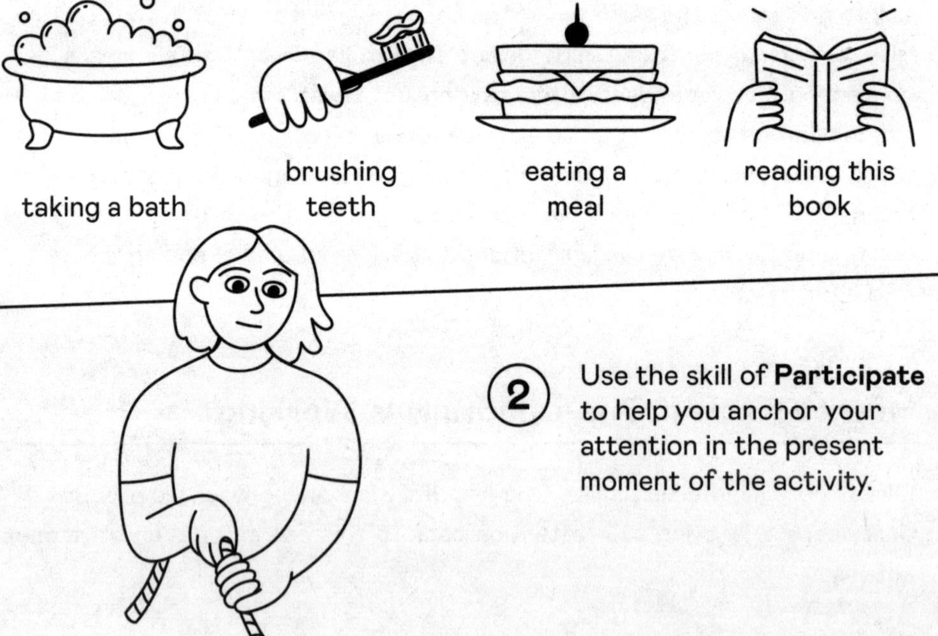

2. Use the skill of **Participate** to help you anchor your attention in the present moment of the activity.

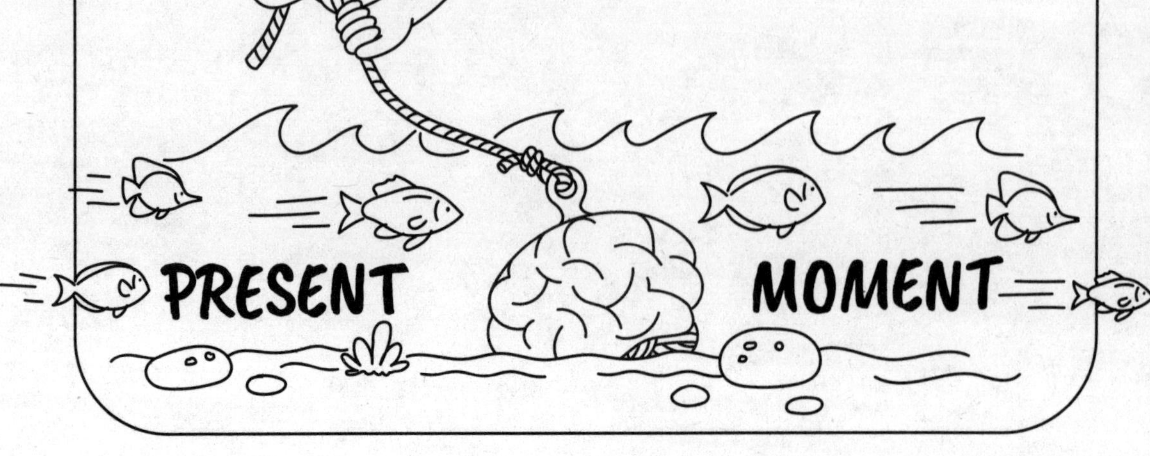

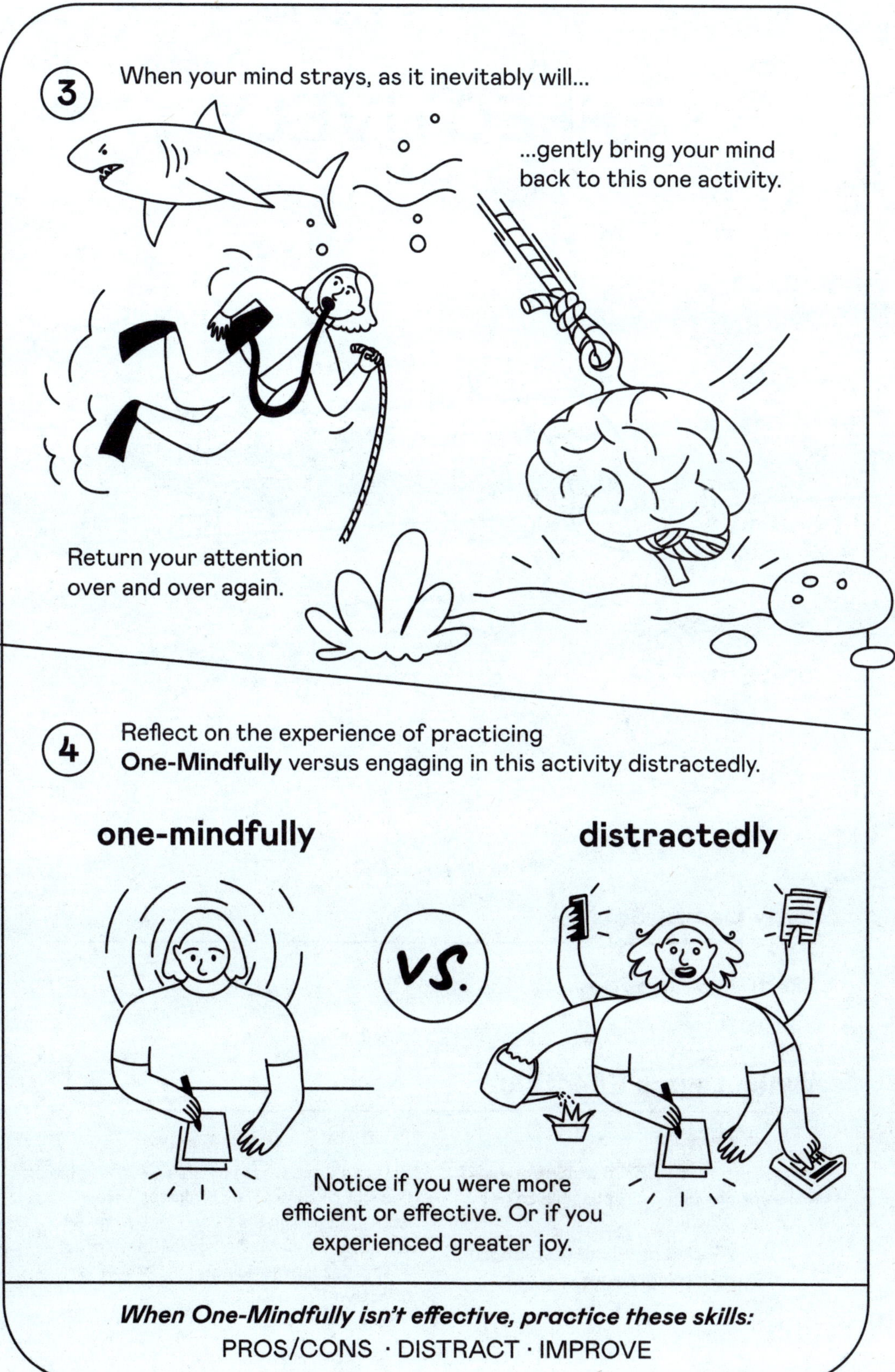
3
When your mind strays, as it inevitably will...
...gently bring your mind back to this one activity.
Return your attention over and over again.
4
Reflect on the experience of practicing **One-Mindfully** versus engaging in this activity distractedly.
one-mindfully
vs.
distractedly
Notice if you were more efficient or effective. Or if you experienced greater joy.
When One-Mindfully isn't effective, practice these skills:
PROS/CONS · DISTRACT · IMPROVE

EFFECTIVELY

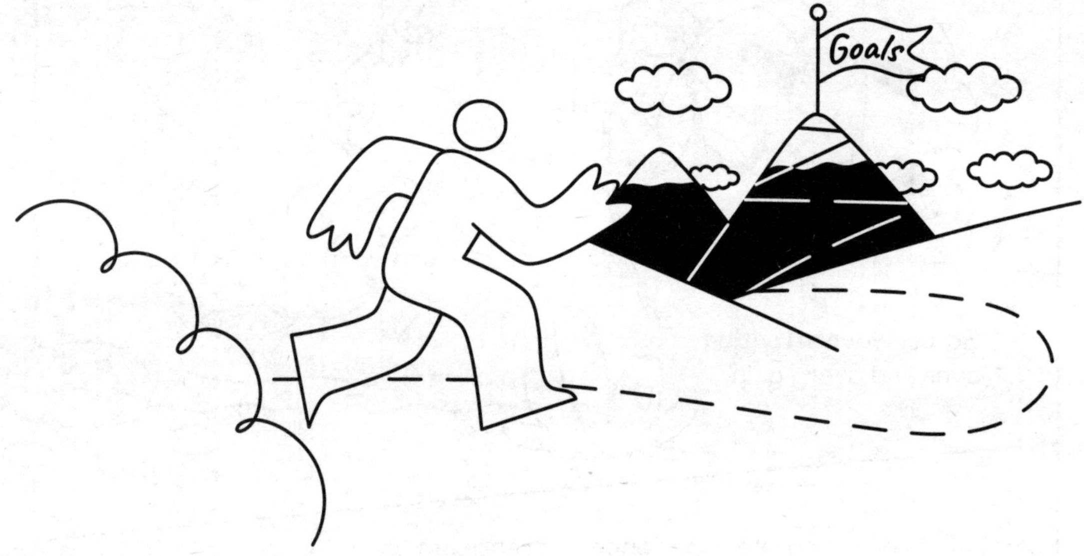

Why Use Effectively?

Effectively gets you closer to your goals!

When to Use Effectively

☑ **Use when:**

- You're in a situation in which you need to act as skillfully as possible to get what you want.
- You are feeling particularly stubborn about something in a way that's not helpful.

☒ **Do NOT use when:**

You can't get what you want. Although the skill of Effectively is almost always useful, sometimes we can't get what we want, no matter how skillful we are. In this case, practicing another skill is effective!

EFFECTIVELY is considered a mindfulness "How" skill, which means it's *how* you practice the other mindfulness skills. Effectively can also be used outside the context of mindfulness exercises and activities. It refers to skillfully doing what's needed in the moment, with your end goal or values in mind.

We often get caught up in being "right" instead of effective. The skill of Effectively means choosing to act effectively even if it means giving up being "right." Effectively is frequently referred to as "doing what works."

For example, imagine that you are at a store and standing in a really long checkout line. You might believe that the people who work there are at fault and think: "*There's no good reason why this line is so long. They should be better at their jobs!*" You might even have a tantrum or voice your displeasure as soon as you make it to the front of the line. But doing so probably only prolongs the time you spend there or keeps you from getting what you want. Practicing Effectively might mean letting go of judgments and accepting the long line so that you can get to your goal as quickly as possible. Or it might mean making different choices the next time you have to go there—arriving at a less busy time or bringing a book with you.

Another example: You have a milestone birthday coming up and you want people to throw you a big party. Rather than waiting for other people to read your mind and give you what you want without you asking, you might realize that acting Effectively here is planning the party yourself *or* asking directly for someone else to take charge. Even if you think this isn't "right," doing so will more likely lead to you having a great party.

How to Know If Effectively Is Working

Effectively is working when you let go of being right and move closer to a goal, in the short term or long term.

How to: Effectively

1. Determine what your goals are in the situation.

2. Identify how you would need to act, communicate, feel, or think to achieve your goals.

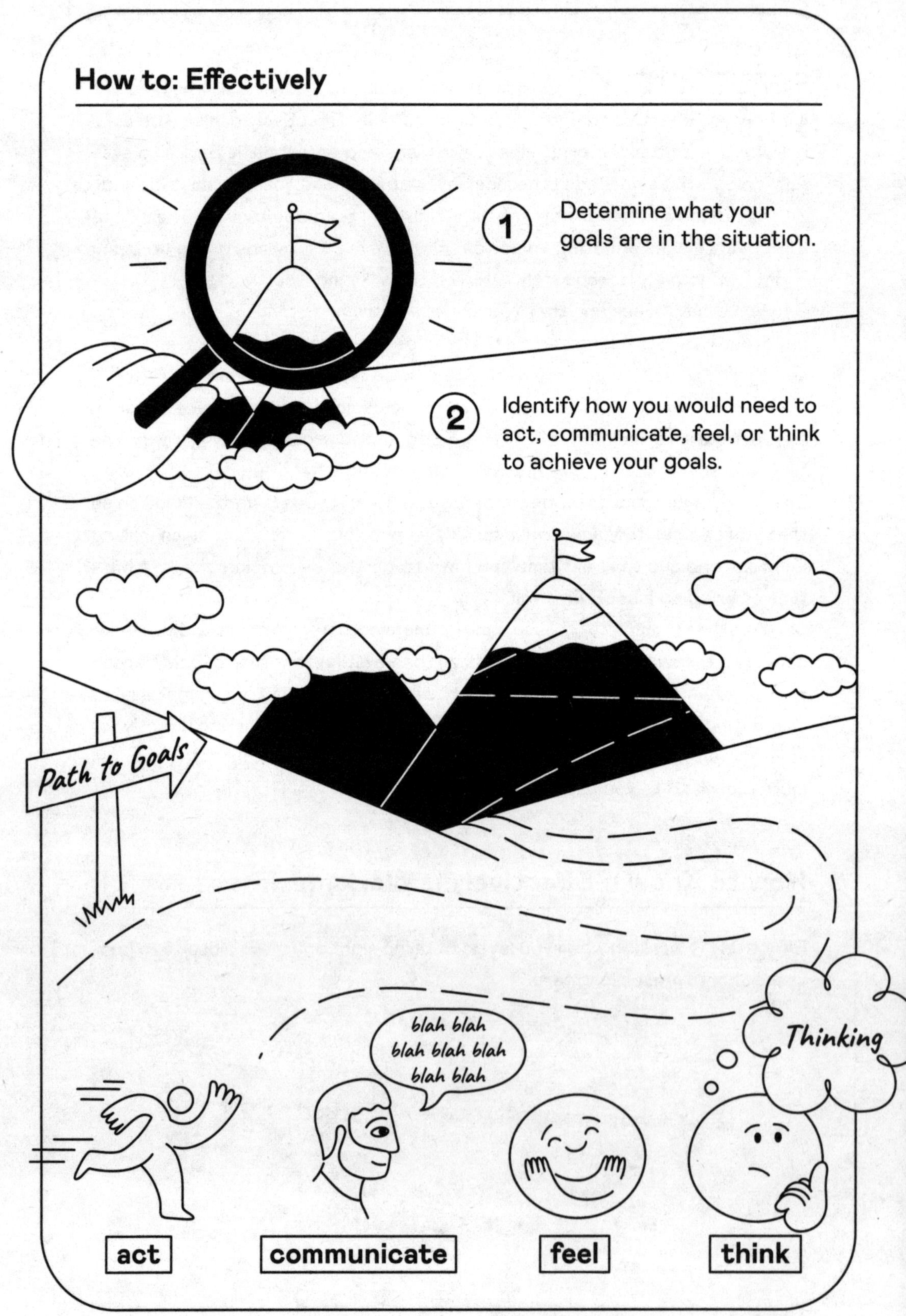

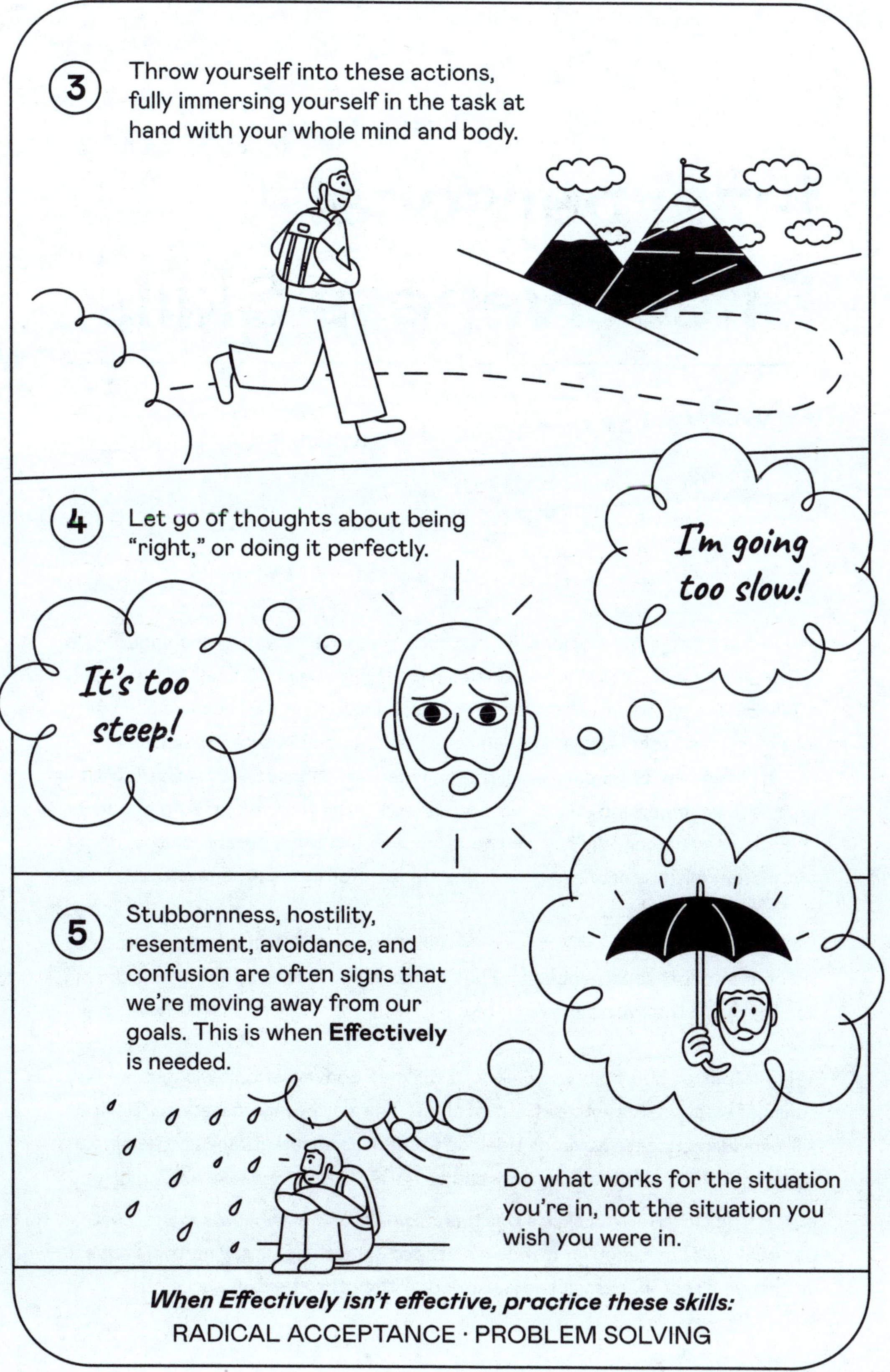

3 Throw yourself into these actions, fully immersing yourself in the task at hand with your whole mind and body.

4 Let go of thoughts about being "right," or doing it perfectly.

5 Stubbornness, hostility, resentment, avoidance, and confusion are often signs that we're moving away from our goals. This is when **Effectively** is needed.

Do what works for the situation you're in, not the situation you wish you were in.

When Effectively isn't effective, practice these skills:

RADICAL ACCEPTANCE · PROBLEM SOLVING

Interpersonal Effectiveness Skills

AN OVERVIEW

There have been low moments in our lives when we have had the thought "if only I didn't have to deal with people, everything would be fine!" It's probably a familiar feeling for most people, yet it is unrealistic. Our lives are filled with interpersonal exchanges, and even relatively benign ones can haunt us afterward. How many of us can recall a time when we behaved ineffectively with a complete stranger and still think about it months or years later? And of course the stakes are generally higher the more we care for a person or the longer our history with someone is. The opportunities for interpersonal situations to go badly seem endless.

The interpersonal effectiveness skills that we teach you here will not get rid of all interpersonal problems. That's impossible. However, they will increase the likelihood that you behave more effectively with others. Here's how.

- Most of the time we walk into difficult conversations without a clear sense of what we hope to get out of them. The skill of Interpersonal Priorities will provide concrete ways for thinking about this ahead of time and helping us determine our goals for a conversation.
- The DEAR MAN skill is designed to help us get what we want (that is, our objective) by teaching us how to ask for something or say no to a request in a manner that increases the likelihood of the other person agreeing.

• The GIVE skill includes strategies for keeping or enhancing the relationship with the other person while we ask for what we want.

• The FAST skill includes strategies for keeping or enhancing our self-respect while we ask for what we want.

• Validation strategies provide you with concrete ways to express acknowledgment and understanding of others. In turn, these strategies will help increase the strength of your relationships and your effectiveness in interpersonal situations. As a bonus, you can use these strategies to validate yourself!

All together, these are a powerful set of tools for our interactions with others, especially ones that feel more high stakes.

Before we dive into those skills, here are a couple more notes. Some people, when first learning these skills, have a reaction something like "I don't like this. It feels like you're teaching me how to be a slick salesperson." The truth is, practicing these skills can feel gimmicky at first until you get more comfortable using them. With practice, you can start to adapt them to your own natural style.

Another common reaction is when people feel that these skills, particularly the DEAR MAN skill, don't fit with their culture or how they were raised. For example, someone might say "In my culture, it is not appropriate to ask an elder so directly for something." That's OK. See if there is anything within these skills that could still work for you.

There is no 100% guarantee with these skills. Sometimes, no matter how skillful we are, we still don't get what we want. That said, with practice, these skills can become extremely effective ways for interacting with others. I (Shireen) confess to still writing out a DEAR MAN script prior to an anticipated difficult conversation—25 years after learning these skills for the first time. That preparatory work never fails to make a difference.

INTERPERSONAL PRIORITIES

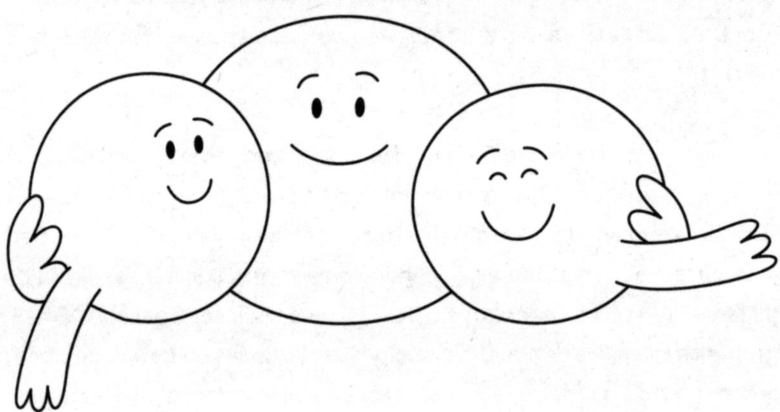

Why Use Interpersonal Priorities?

Figuring out your Interpersonal Priorities is essential for increasing your effectiveness in difficult interpersonal conversations.

When to Use Interpersonal Priorities

☑ **Use when:**

- You are not totally clear about what you want out of an interaction.
- You are anticipating a difficult conversation.
- You are experiencing anxiety about asking for something or saying no to something.

☒ **Do NOT use when:**

The interpersonal situation is a very minor one—you don't want to obsess over every interaction with someone.

INTERPERSONAL PRIORITIES is a key process to engage in before you have a difficult or high-stakes conversation with someone. When things go badly in a conversation with another person, it's often because we were unclear ahead of time about what we were looking for in that conversation. Interpersonal Priorities consist of three ranked elements: meeting your objective, keeping (or enhancing) the relationship, and keeping (or enhancing) your self-respect.

The skill involves asking yourself three questions about your Interpersonal Priorities, then ranking them in order.

1. What do I want to get out of this interaction? (This is your objective.)
2. How do I want the other person to feel about it or me after the interaction? (This is the relationship.)
3. How do I want to feel about myself after the interaction? (This is your self-respect.)

Once you know the answers to these questions, you put them in order of importance *for this particular interaction.* Knowing how you would rank these three priorities prior to the conversation will aid you in acting most effectively for the situation.

How to Know If Interpersonal Priorities Are Working

Determining your Interpersonal Priorities will help guide you in effectively using other interpersonal skills, like DEAR MAN, GIVE, and FAST. However, sometimes just being clear about these priorities is enough to navigate a situation effectively.

How to: Interpersonal Priorities

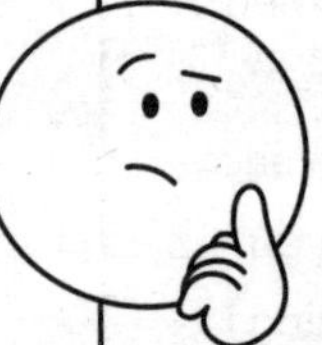

(1) Before going into an important conversation, ask yourself three questions:

OBJECTIVE

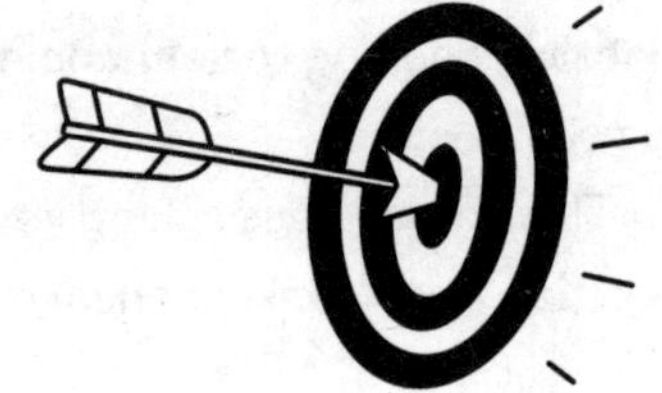

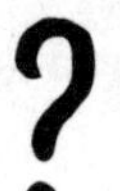

What is my objective in this situation – what am I hoping to get out of it?

Come up with an objective that is observable and achievable.

"I want the other person to appreciate me" is *NOT* a helpful objective since you can't truly know what another person feels. Consider something concrete like "I want this person to agree to help me with this task."

RELATIONSHIP

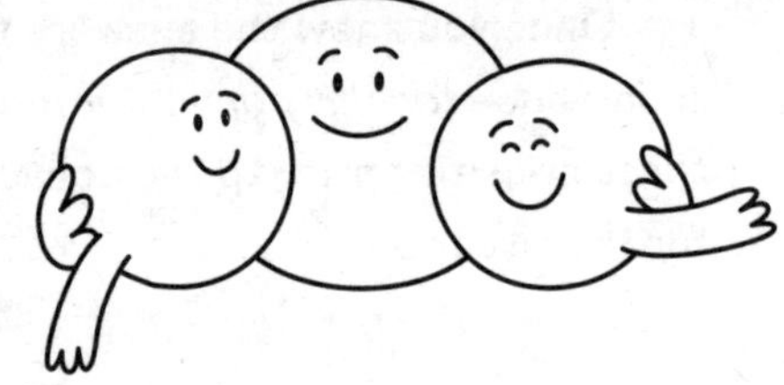

How do I want the other person to feel about me as a result of this conversation?

The default answer to this question tends to be "I want this person to like me!"

Consider the nature of the relationship (stranger vs. close friend), the short and long-term relationship goals, and how important it is (or isn't) to act in accordance with them.

SELF-RESPECT

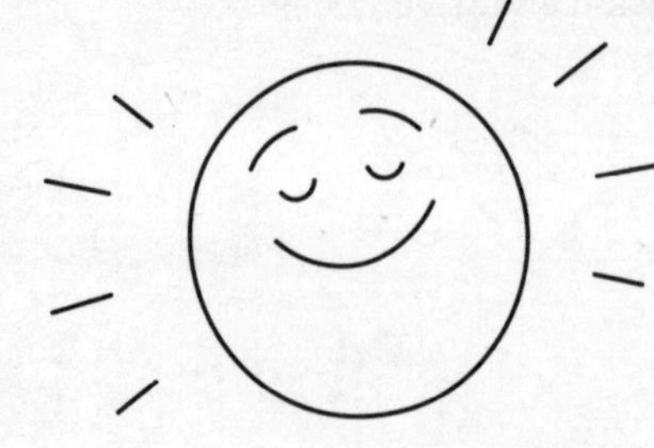

How do I want to feel about myself as a result of this conversation?

The default answer is usually "I want to feel good about myself!"

Consider your values and your beliefs and how important it is (or isn't) to act in accordance with them.

(2) Once you have answers to all three of your questions, rank them in order of priority. Put objective, relationship, and self-respect in order of importance for this particular interaction.

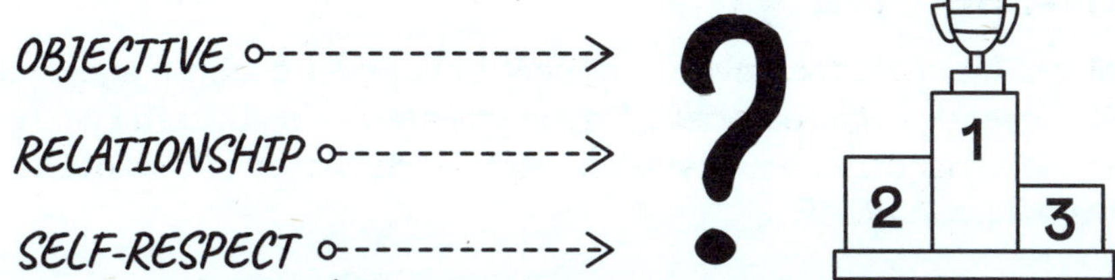

Sometimes ranking these three elements is enough to provide an "aha" moment about how to move forward.

But if you're still unsure, having them ranked will help you apply the other interpersonal effectiveness skills.

(3) Over time, notice if there are patterns in your rankings.

If you tend to rank things the same way, you might be stuck in unhelpful interpersonal habits.

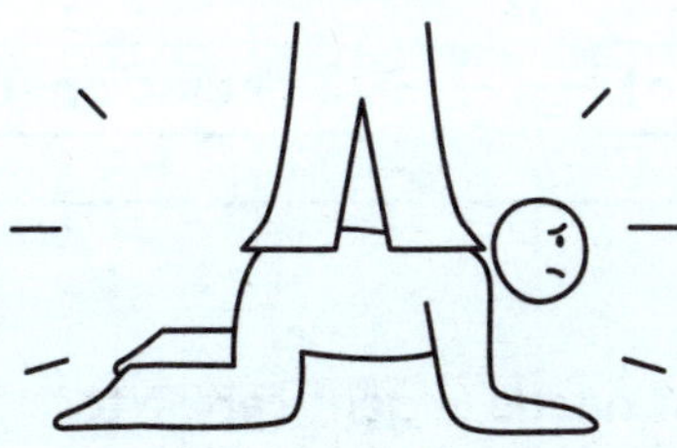

Do you always put relationship first, which means longer-term damage to your self-respect?

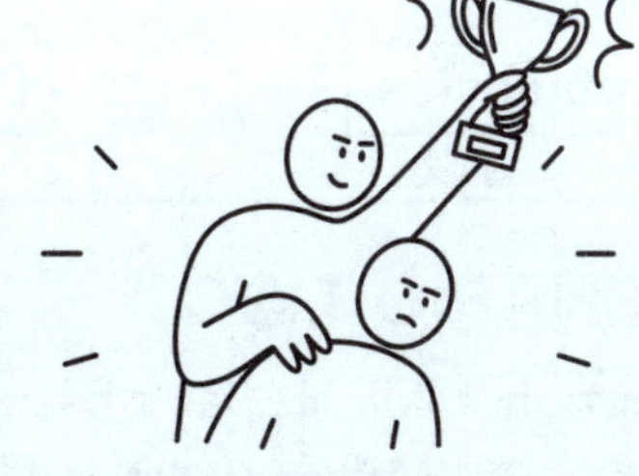

Do you always prioritize objectives and lose relationships as a result?

Consider the short-term and long-term impact of your rankings. Use **Wise Mind** (page 18) to help determine whether your priority rankings are most effective.

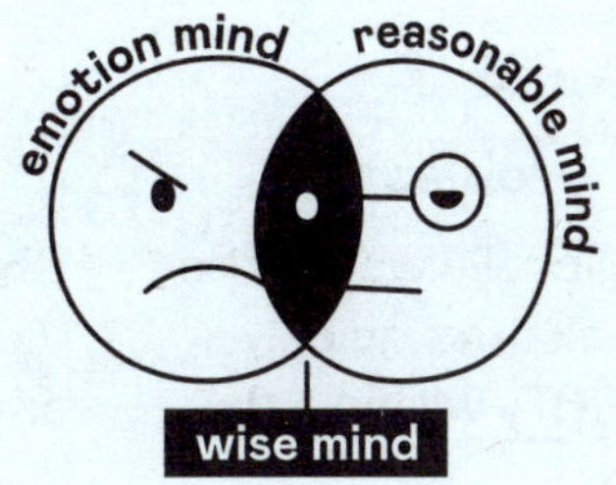

When Interpersonal Priorities are hard to determine, practice these skills:

WISE MIND · PROS/CONS

In Practice: Interpersonal Priorities

SCENARIO ONE

Situation: Alex paid for Devon's concert ticket over a month ago, and despite several polite reminders, Devon still hasn't reimbursed him. Alex values their friendship but is starting to feel frustrated and wants to resolve the issue ASAP.

Goals:

objective	relationship	self-respect
Get Devon to pay the money owed for the concert ticket.	Maintain a positive and respectful friendship with Devon.	Feel proud about doing something that is hard for him.
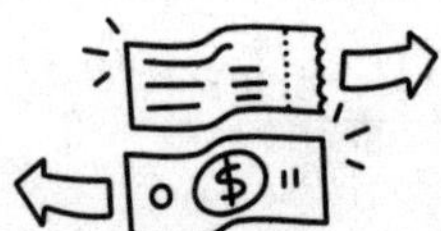	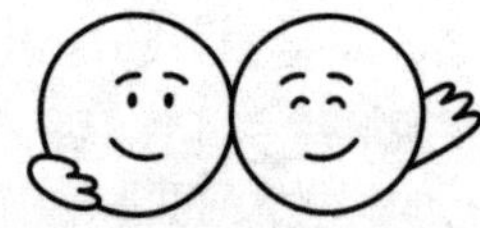	

Wise Mind Decision: Alex prioritizes getting his money back, even if it causes some tension. Standing up for himself and setting limits matters, and he's willing to risk awkwardness to resolve the issue.

Priority Ranking:

1 objective --------> 2 self-respect ------> 3 relationship

SCENARIO TWO

Situation: Michelle has a bathroom leak that needs urgent repair to prevent permanent damage. Her landlord, Wanda, isn't great with maintenance, but Michelle wants to stay on Wanda's good side to keep her rent low.

Goals:

objective	relationship	self-respect
Michelle wants the leak fixed quickly—ideally within a day.	She wants her landlord to view her as a responsible and grateful tenant.	She wants to feel like she is appropriately assertive.
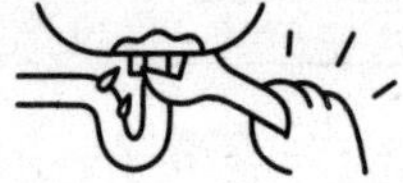	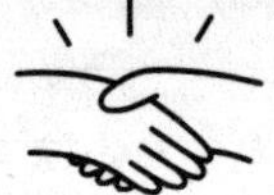	

Wise Mind Decision: Michelle prioritizes keeping her landlord happy since cheap rent is worth it. She's willing to compromise her self-respect, exaggerating the issue or acting helpless if it speeds up the repair.

Priority Ranking:

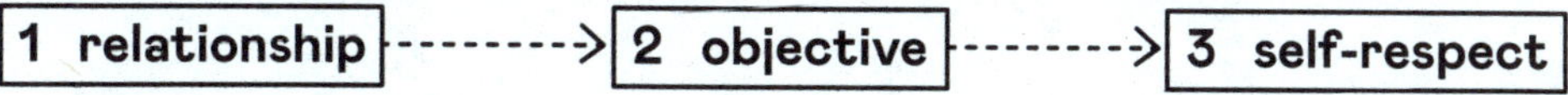

SCENARIO THREE

Situation: Charlie's aunt frequently comments on their appearance at family gatherings, making them feel uncomfortable and self-conscious. This is especially tough during holiday dinners when Charlie just wants to enjoy time with family. They've decided it's time to speak up and address the issue directly.

Goals:

objective

Get their aunt to stop making comments about their appearance.

relationship

Maintain a positive family relationship and for their aunt to view them as respectful.

self-respect

Feel proud for standing up for themselves.

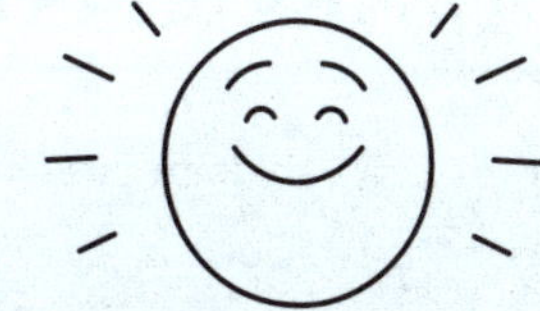

Wise Mind Decision: Charlie prioritizes self-respect while hoping to maintain family bonds and put an end to their aunt's comments. They understand that clear assertion may cause temporary tension, but they're willing to take that risk.

Priority Ranking:

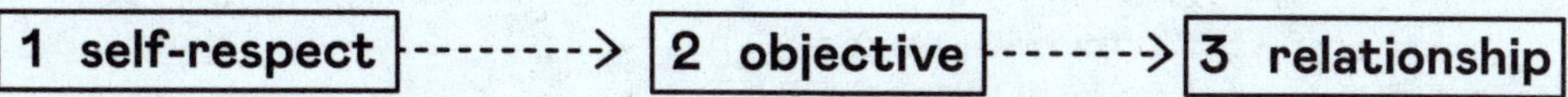

Note that you might have different rankings for these examples—that's the point! There is no "right" answer.

DEAR MAN

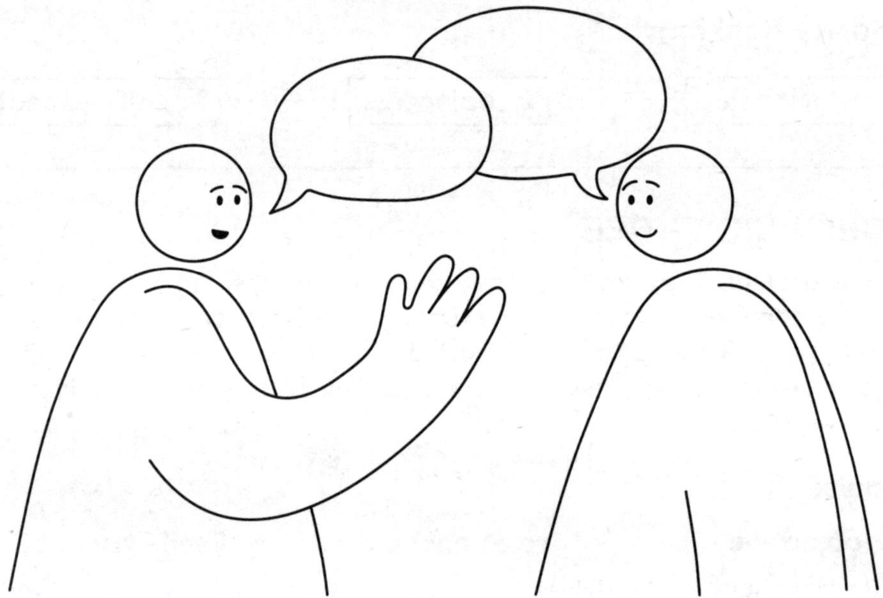

Why Use DEAR MAN?

DEAR MAN improves the likelihood that you'll get your objective in interpersonal situations.

When to Use DEAR MAN

☑ **Use when:**

- You want something or want to say no, and
- You know, based on doing some homework first, that the other person can give you what you want and that it's a good time to make the request, and
- You have ranked getting your objective as most important in your Interpersonal Priorities.

☒ **Do NOT use when:**

- You don't know what you want.
- The other person can't give you what you want.
- You are feeling too dysregulated to ask effectively.

DEAR MAN is an acronym for a set of steps designed for situations when you are asking for something or saying no to something. This skill helps you communicate in a manner that increases the likelihood of success. Generally speaking, the DEAR parts are what you say when making the request and the MAN parts are how you engage in the conversation.

- D Describe: Describe the situation that is prompting this request. Describe just the facts!
- E Express: Express your thoughts and opinions about the situation. Use "I" statements.
- A Assert: Very explicitly and specifically ask for what you want or state what you are saying no to. Do not beat around the bush or assume the other person can guess.
- R Reinforce: Let the other person know what good thing will come their way if they agree to your request. This could be sincerely saying "I'd greatly appreciate it if you did this for me" or "In return, I'll take you out for coffee." (Be sure to follow through!)
- M (stay) Mindful: Keep focused on your objective and don't get steered off track (by yourself or the other person).
- A Appear confident: Notice it's "appear" confident, not "be" confident. Make eye contact, use a confident voice tone, stand up straight.
- N Negotiate: If the other person is not acceding to your request, ask for other solutions to the problem. Be willing to give something in order to get something you want.

DEAR MAN requires practice and planning. When you know you have a difficult conversation coming up, putting aside time to think about and plan for it is essential.

How to Know If DEAR MAN Is Working

If you ask for something and the other person says yes or is willing to negotiate with you on a preferred outcome, or you say no to a request and the other person accepts it.

How to: DEAR MAN

1. Use **Interpersonal Priorities** rankings to determine how strongly to emphasize **DEAR MAN** for achieving your objective.

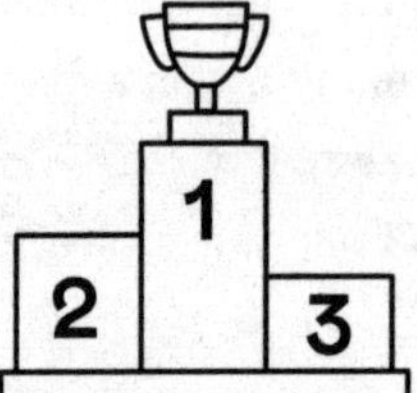

for example

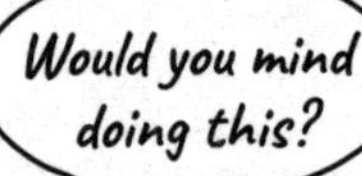

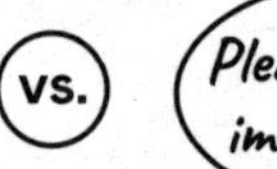

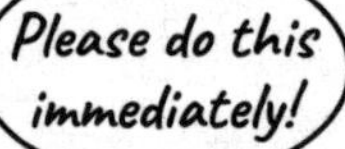

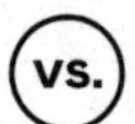

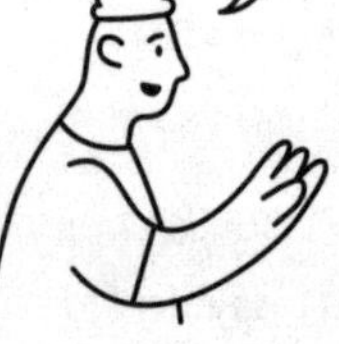
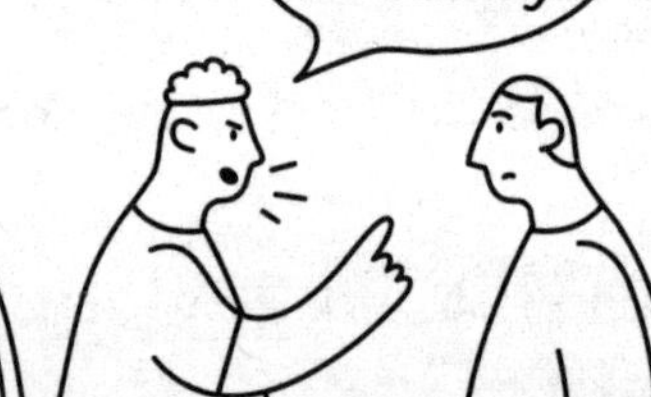
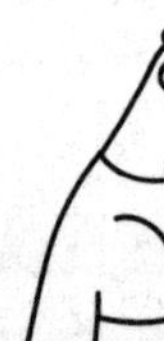
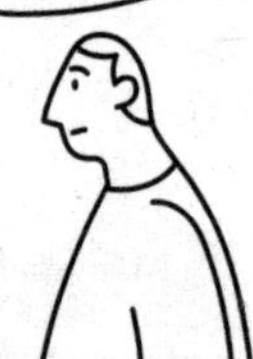

2. If possible, prepare your **D-E-A-R** ahead of time. Try to keep each statement as brief as possible.

 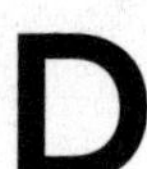 **Describe** the situation.

DO: Describe just the facts. Keep it brief.

DON'T: Add on interpretations or judgments.

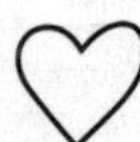 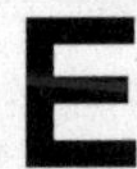 **Express** your thoughts and feelings.

DO: Use "I" statements ("I feel...").

DON'T: Say "you should," moralize, or accuse.

 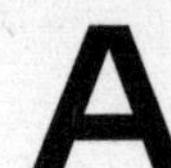 **Assert** what you want.

DO: Ask or say "no" directly.

DON'T: Hedge or assume others can read your mind.

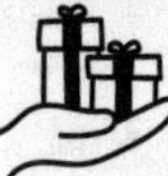 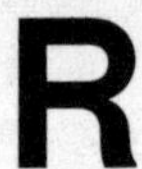 **Reinforce** by telling them what they'll gain by agreeing.

DO: Be specific. Follow through.

DON'T: Over-promise. Flake out.

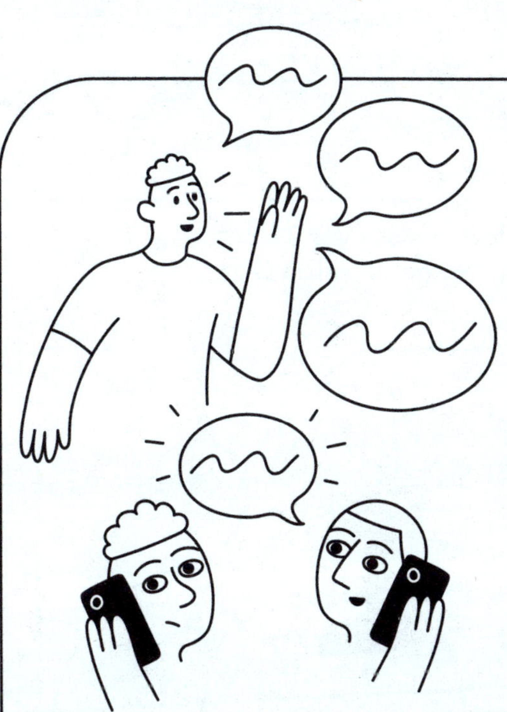

3 Practice saying the **D-E-A-R** steps out loud.

TRY THIS

Listen to how your request sounds and make adjustments to be more clear, concise, and confident sounding.

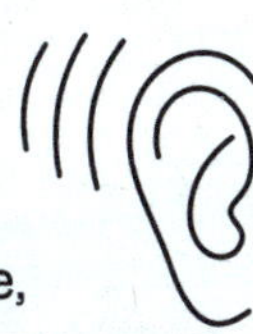

Consider asking a friend to practice with you and provide feedback.

4 When delivering your **D-E-A-R** remember the **M-A-N**.

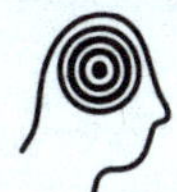

M **(stay) Mindful** of your goals in the situation.

DO: Be a broken record. Repeat your **assert** over and over.

DON'T: Respond to attacks, threats, or diversions.

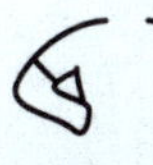

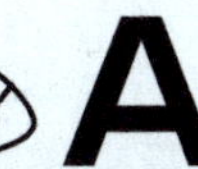

A **Appear confident** while engaging in the conversation.

DO: Maintain eye contact, use a steady voice, and sit or stand with an open posture.

DON'T: Fidget, avoid eye contact, or use a hesitant or apologetic tone.

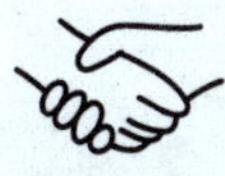

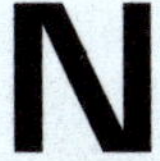

N **Negotiate** to achieve your objectives.

DO: Be willing to give to get. Offer compromises. Engage in collaborative problem solving.

DON'T: Demand everything go your way. Ignore the other person's perspective.

When DEAR MAN isn't effective, practice these skills:

SELF-SOOTHE · RADICAL ACCEPTANCE

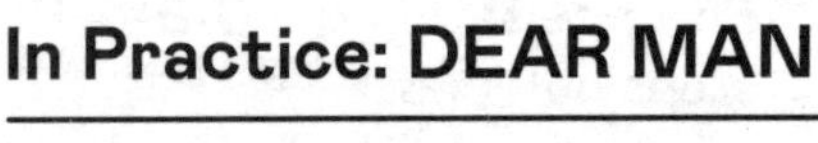

In Practice: DEAR MAN

Meet Alex. Alex paid for Devon's concert ticket over a month ago, but Devon still hasn't paid him back despite repeated reminders.

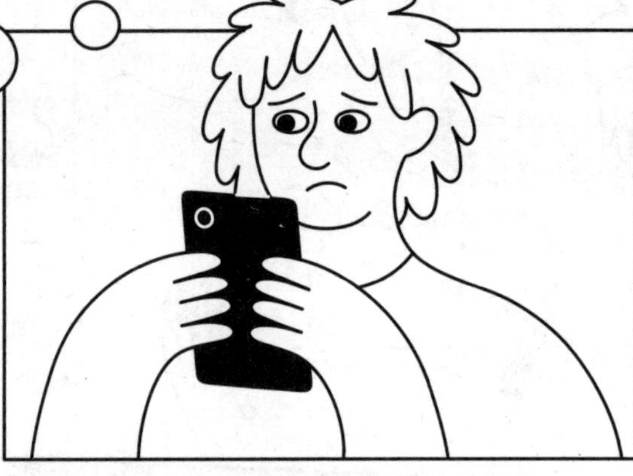

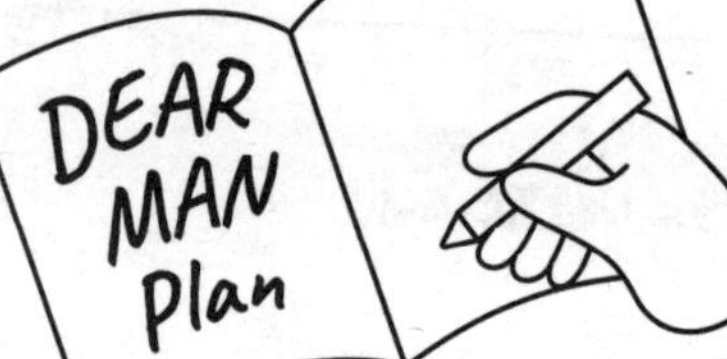

Since Alex's #1 priority is to get reimbursed, he writes out his **DEAR MAN** script to get his money back.

1 Describe

Alex begins with **Describe**, stating the facts.

2 Express

He uses **Express** to share the impact.

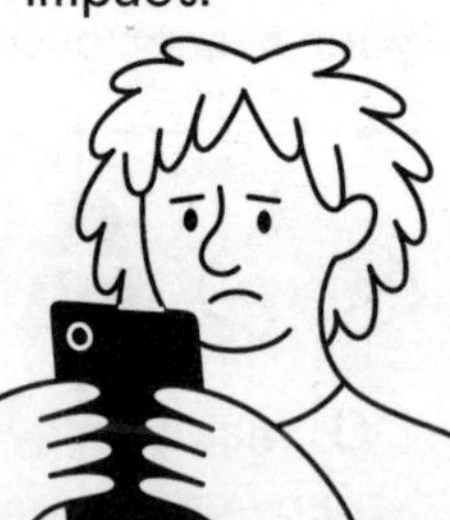

3 Assert

In the **Assert** step, Alex clearly states his request.

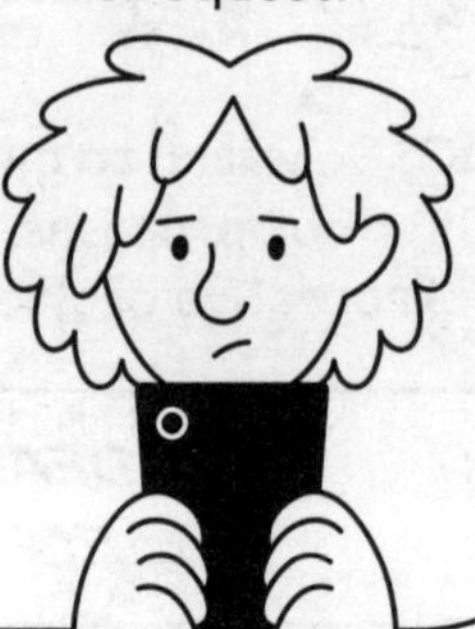

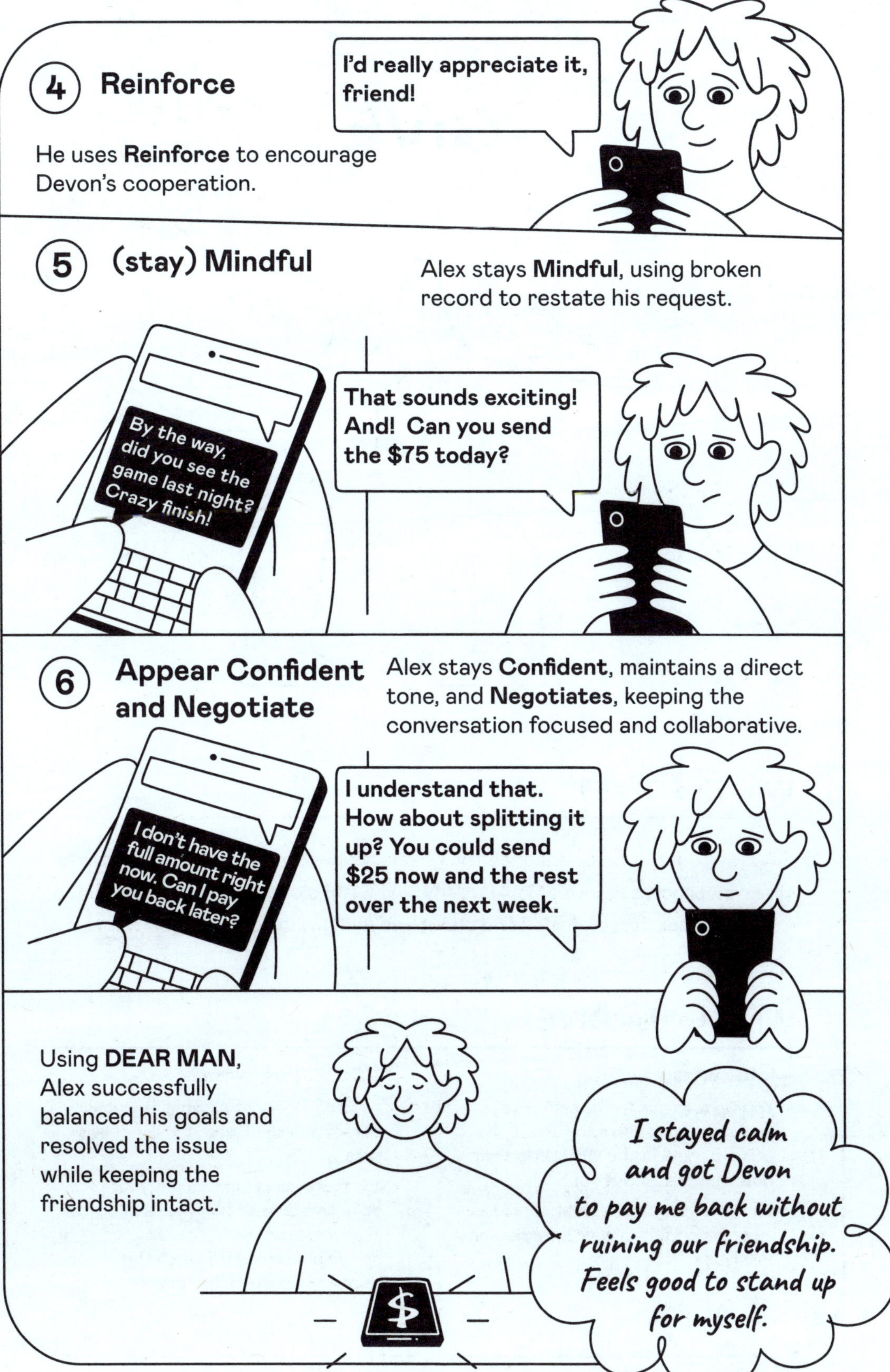

4 Reinforce
I'd really appreciate it, friend!
He uses **Reinforce** to encourage Devon's cooperation.
5 (stay) Mindful
Alex stays **Mindful**, using broken record to restate his request.
By the way, did you see the game last night? Crazy finish!
That sounds exciting! And! Can you send the $75 today?
6 Appear Confident and Negotiate
Alex stays **Confident**, maintains a direct tone, and **Negotiates**, keeping the conversation focused and collaborative.
I don't have the full amount right now. Can I pay you back later?
I understand that. How about splitting it up? You could send $25 now and the rest over the next week.
Using **DEAR MAN**, Alex successfully balanced his goals and resolved the issue while keeping the friendship intact.
I stayed calm and got Devon to pay me back without ruining our friendship. Feels good to stand up for myself.
$

GIVE

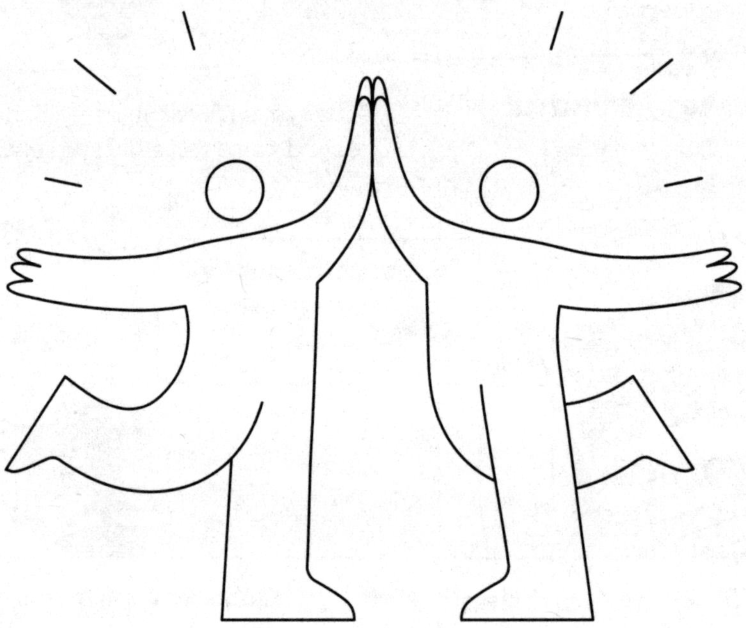

Why Use GIVE?

GIVE helps maintain or enhance the relationship when you ask for something. When incorporated into a DEAR MAN, the GIVE skill increases the likelihood that the other person feels good about you and giving you what you want.

When to Use GIVE

☑ **Use when:**

- You want to ask for or say no to something *and* you care about the other person in the interaction and how they feel about you.
- You have ranked the relationship as most important in your Interpersonal Priorities.

☒ **Do NOT use when:**

- You don't care at all what the other person will think about you. (This is rare.)
- It is more important to get your objective or maintain your self-respect. In other words, do not emphasize GIVE when the relationship isn't a key priority.

GIVE is an acronym for a set of skills to enhance your DEAR MAN interaction. In most interpersonal situations, we want the other person to like us or have a high opinion of us when it's over. The GIVE skills increase the chances that will happen by providing a focus on enhancing or maintaining the relationship. Using these skills can also increase the chances of someone meeting your requests. So, even if you aren't concerned about them liking you, the GIVE skills might still be helpful to use.

- G (be) Gentle: Be gentle by using a kind and respectful tone and behavior. Avoid making threats, judgments, or attacks.
- I (act) Interested: Listen and appear interested in the other person. Do this by facing them, making eye contact, nodding, avoiding interrupting, and using the One-Mindfully skill in the conversation.
- V Validate: State directly how their thoughts, feelings, and/or behaviors make sense and are understandable. Try to see the situation from their perspective and express that.
- E Easy manner: Try to be light and easy, as opposed to overly serious or severe. Consider smiling and using humor.

An important note about the GIVE skills here. Although much of our communication now exists through text messages, the GIVE skills are often more effectively conveyed when the person can see your face or hear your voice. Many times, we use text communication to avoid difficult conversations or the discomfort of someone not liking our request. However, those text conversations often don't lead to our preferred outcomes and are prone to miscommunication. We encourage you to use the GIVE skills "in real life" with someone, especially when the stakes are high.

How to Know If GIVE Is Working

If you and the other person feel good about the relationship when an interpersonal interaction is over.

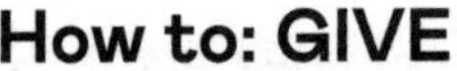

How to: GIVE

1. To apply **GIVE** means to deliver your **DEAR MAN** while prioritizing the relationship.

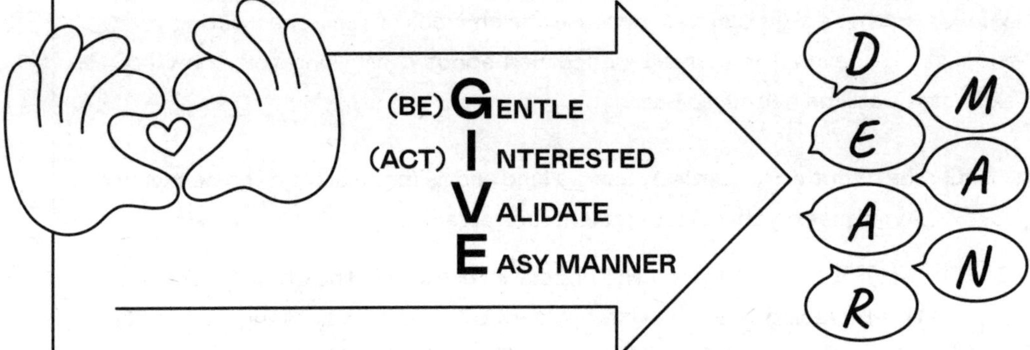

2. **Gentle.** Be respectful in your:

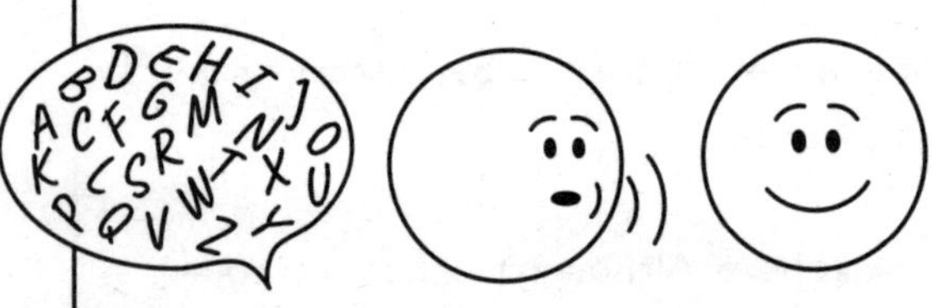

words voice tone expression

Stay in the conversation gracefully even if it's painful.

Don't threaten, judge, or walk away.

3. **(act) Interested.**

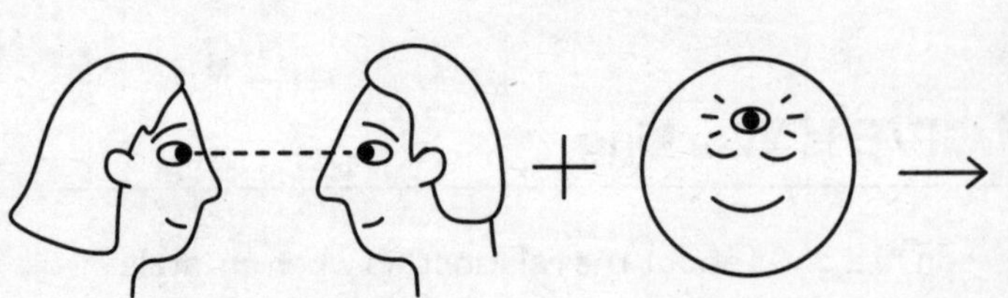

Maintain good eye contact. + Use **One-Mindfully**. → To let the other person know that you are paying attention.

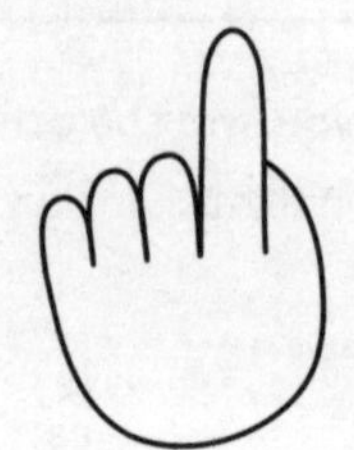

4 **Validate.** Let the other person know that their...

thoughts **feelings** **behaviors** make sense given their past or current experience.

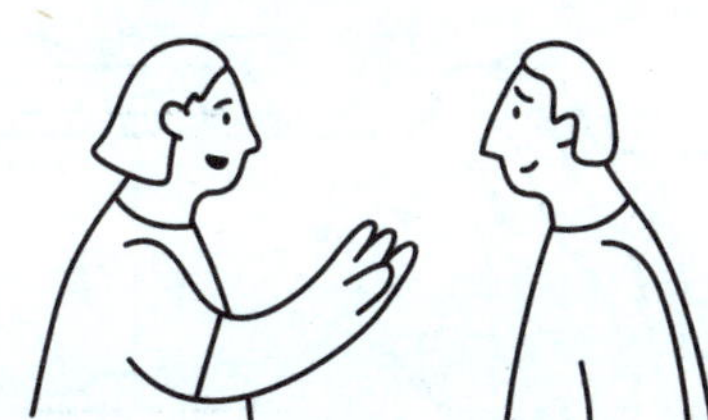

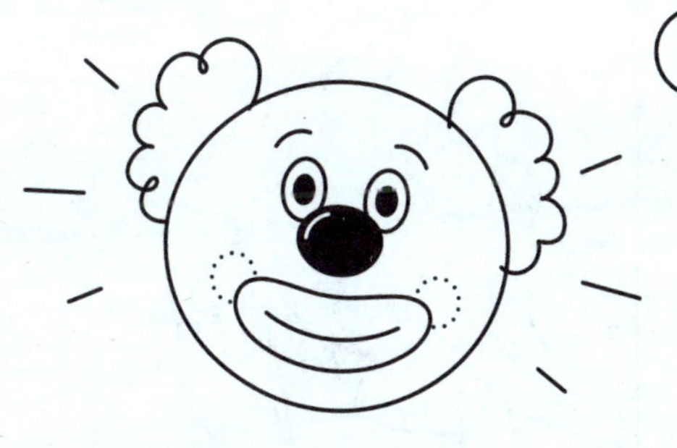

5 **Easy manner.** Think about how you can lighten up the intensity of the conversation and add humor if appropriate.

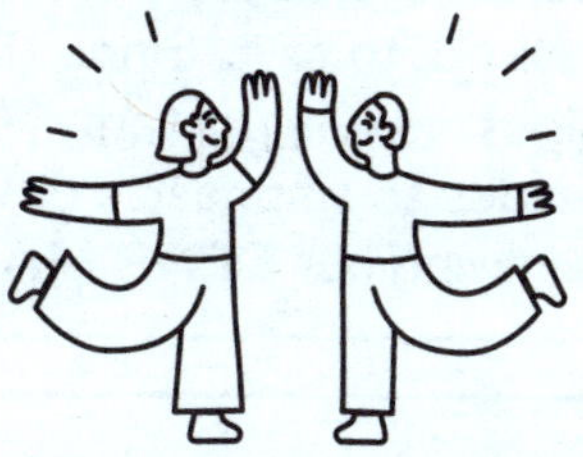

Be polite and kind instead of confrontational and intense.

Remember the adage "you attract more flies with honey than with vinegar."

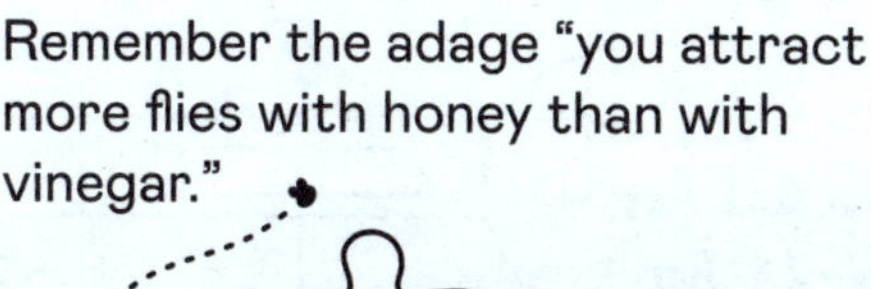

AND

6 Ask someone to role-play with you so that you can practice all these elements in advance.

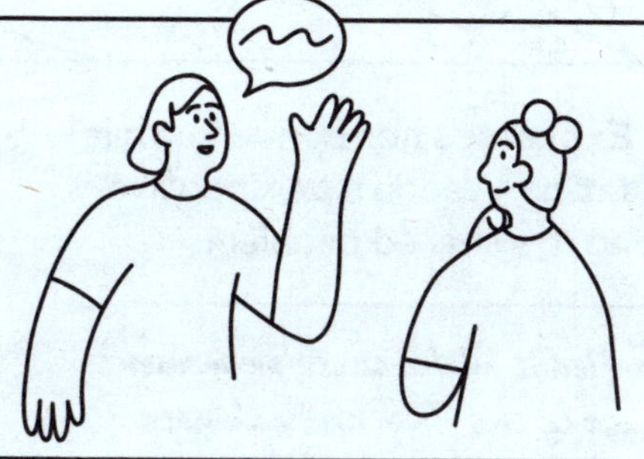

When GIVE isn't effective, practice these skills:

SELF-SOOTHE · RADICAL ACCEPTANCE

In Practice: GIVE

Meet Michelle.

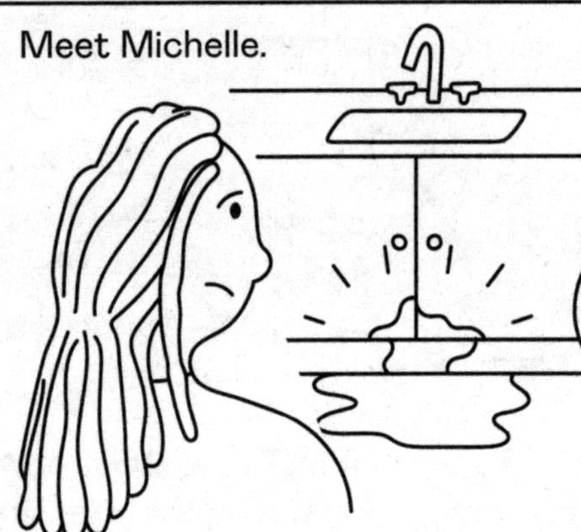

Michelle has a water leak in her kitchen and needs Wanda, her landlord, to fix it. Since the relationship is most important, Michelle decides to emphasize **GIVE** while delivering her **DEAR MAN**.

Michelle begins with **Easy manner**, setting a friendly tone for the conversation.

1 Describe and Express

Michelle uses **(be) Gentle** to describe the issue without blaming or criticizing Wanda.

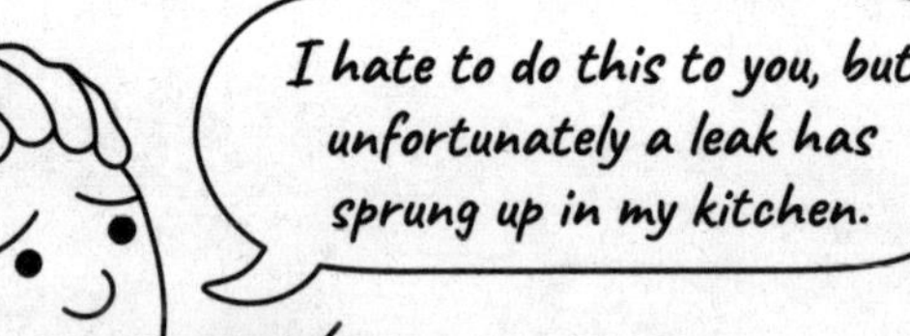

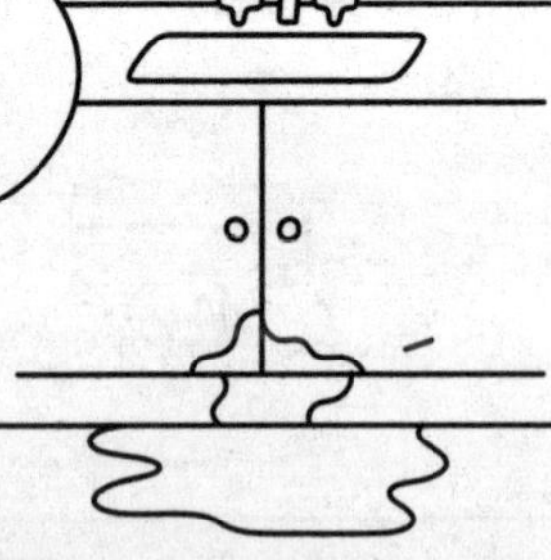

She **Expresses** her concern while **Validating** Wanda's perspective, making it a shared problem.

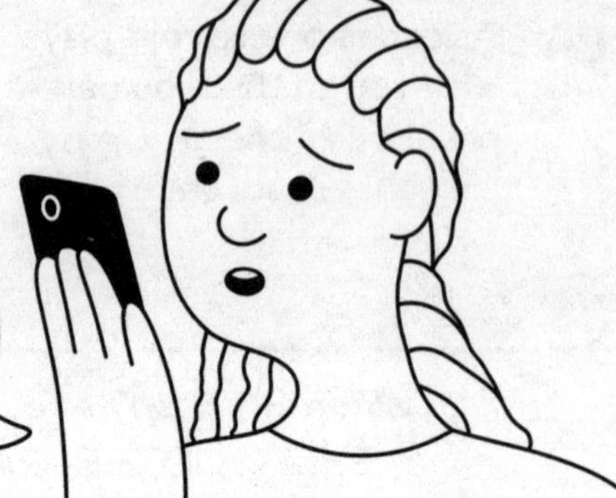

2 Assert and Reinforce

Michelle **Asserts** her request clearly while keeping her tone **Gentle** and **Reinforcing** the mutual benefit of fixing the leak promptly.

Would you mind calling a repairperson and have them come over right away to fix it?

You know how well I take care of this apartment, and I'd love for it to stay in great shape for me and for you!

3 (act) Interested

Wanda starts to push back, getting distracted by her busy day.

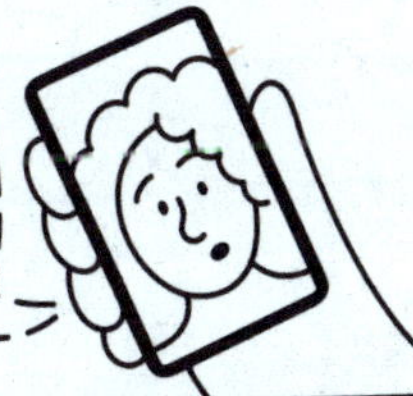

Michelle acts **Interested**, listening actively without interrupting Wanda.

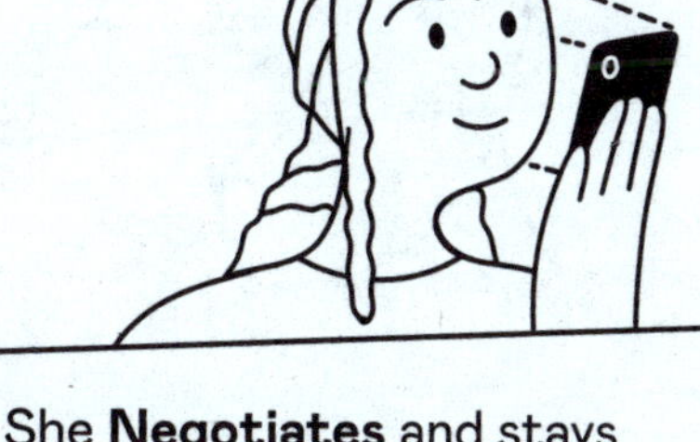

4 Validate

Michelle **Validates** Wanda's feelings.

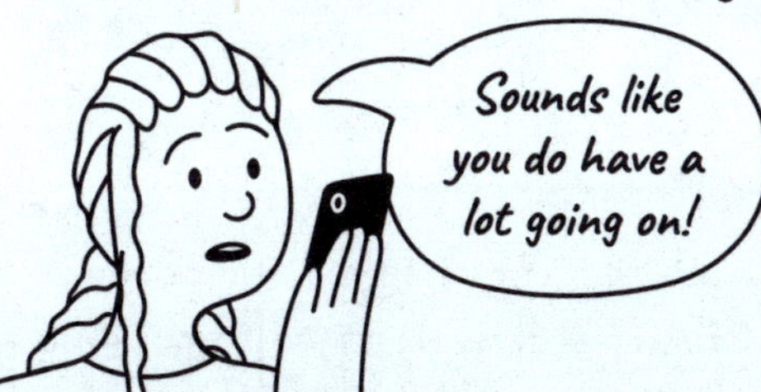

She **Negotiates** and stays **Mindful**, focusing on her goal while proposing a solution that helps Wanda while reinforcing the need for quick action.

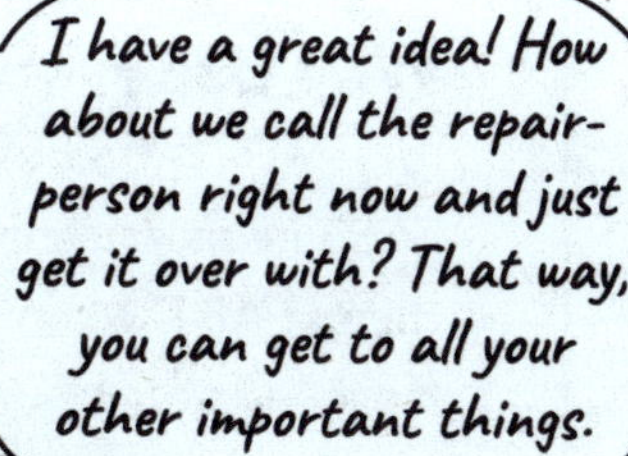

Wanda agrees to make the call, thanks to Michelle's use of **GIVE**.

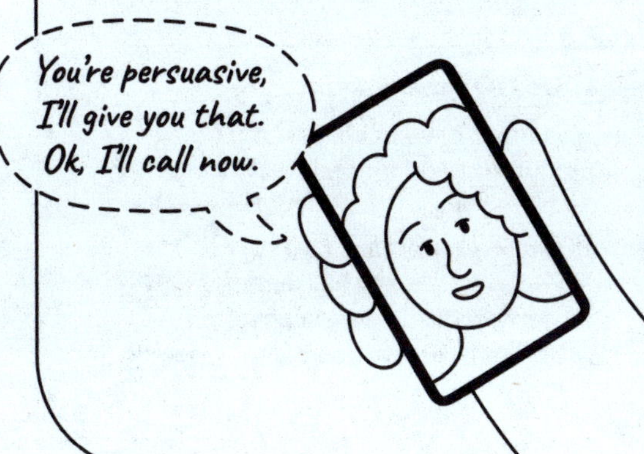

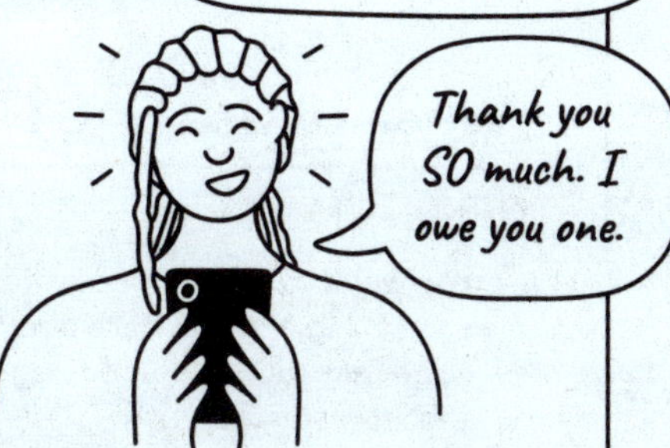

Michelle ends with **Reinforcement**, showing appreciation and strengthening the relationship for the future.

FAST

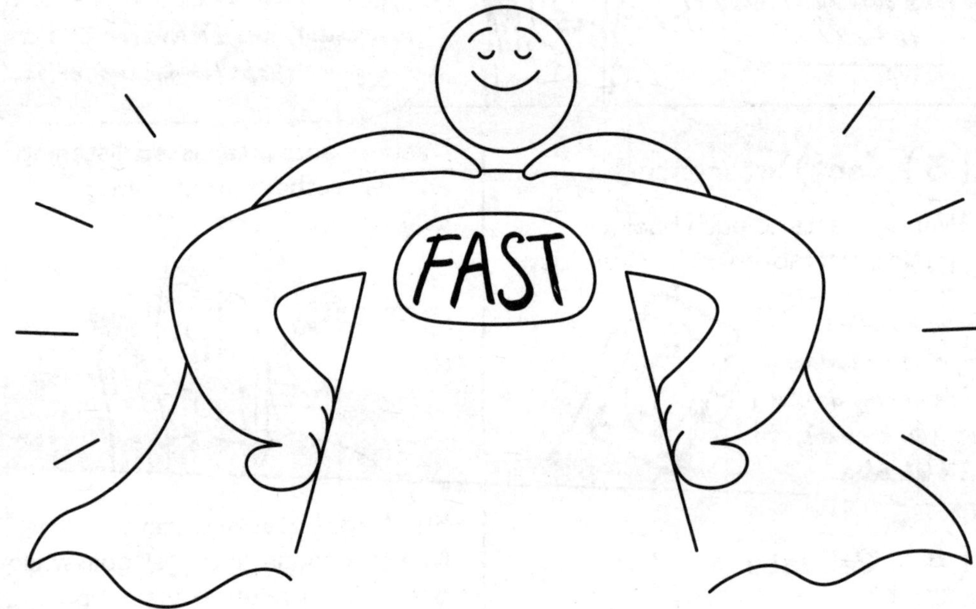

Why Use FAST?

FAST helps you enhance or maintain your self-respect when you ask for something. FAST, when incorporated into a DEAR MAN, is designed to help you feel good about how you tried to get your objective.

When to Use FAST

☑ **Use when:**

- You want to ask for or say no to something and you care about how you'll feel about yourself regarding the interaction.
- You have ranked self-respect as most important in your Interpersonal Priorities.

☒ **Do NOT use when:**

- You don't care at all how you feel about yourself in the interaction. (This is rare.)
- It is more important to get your objective or keep the relationship. In other words, do not emphasize FAST when self-respect isn't a key priority.

FAST is an acronym for a set of skills to enhance your DEAR MAN interaction by focusing on your self-respect. Incorporating these skills into your DEAR MAN will increase the likelihood that you will feel good about yourself and your actions when the interaction is over.

- F (be) Fair: Be fair to yourself and the other person. Don't ask for more than what is possible. Validate your own feelings and wishes.
- A (no) Apologies: Don't apologize for having an opinion or a desire for something. If you need to apologize for something you did or didn't do, do it once and move on. Don't overapologize. Avoid looking ashamed or guilty about asking for something.
- S Stick to values: Have integrity and stick to your values. Don't give in to something that does not fit your own values. Be clear on what you believe and want.
- T (be) Truthful: Avoid lying. Even "little white lies" can erode your self-respect with time. Don't act helpless or exaggerate to get what you want.

Like the other interpersonal skills, FAST takes practice. It can be especially difficult for those who tend to deprioritize self-respect in the interest of maintaining relationships and keeping other people happy. Some people also never had someone in their life who could model standing up for themselves in ways that were effective. It makes sense that this skill may be particularly hard for some people. Yet, it's important not to overlook the importance of self-respect. If you don't attend to how you feel about yourself, over time your self-respect will erode, impacting your sense of well-being and your effectiveness with others.

How to Know If FAST Is Working

If you ask for or say no to something and you feel good about yourself and how you handled it when the interaction is over.

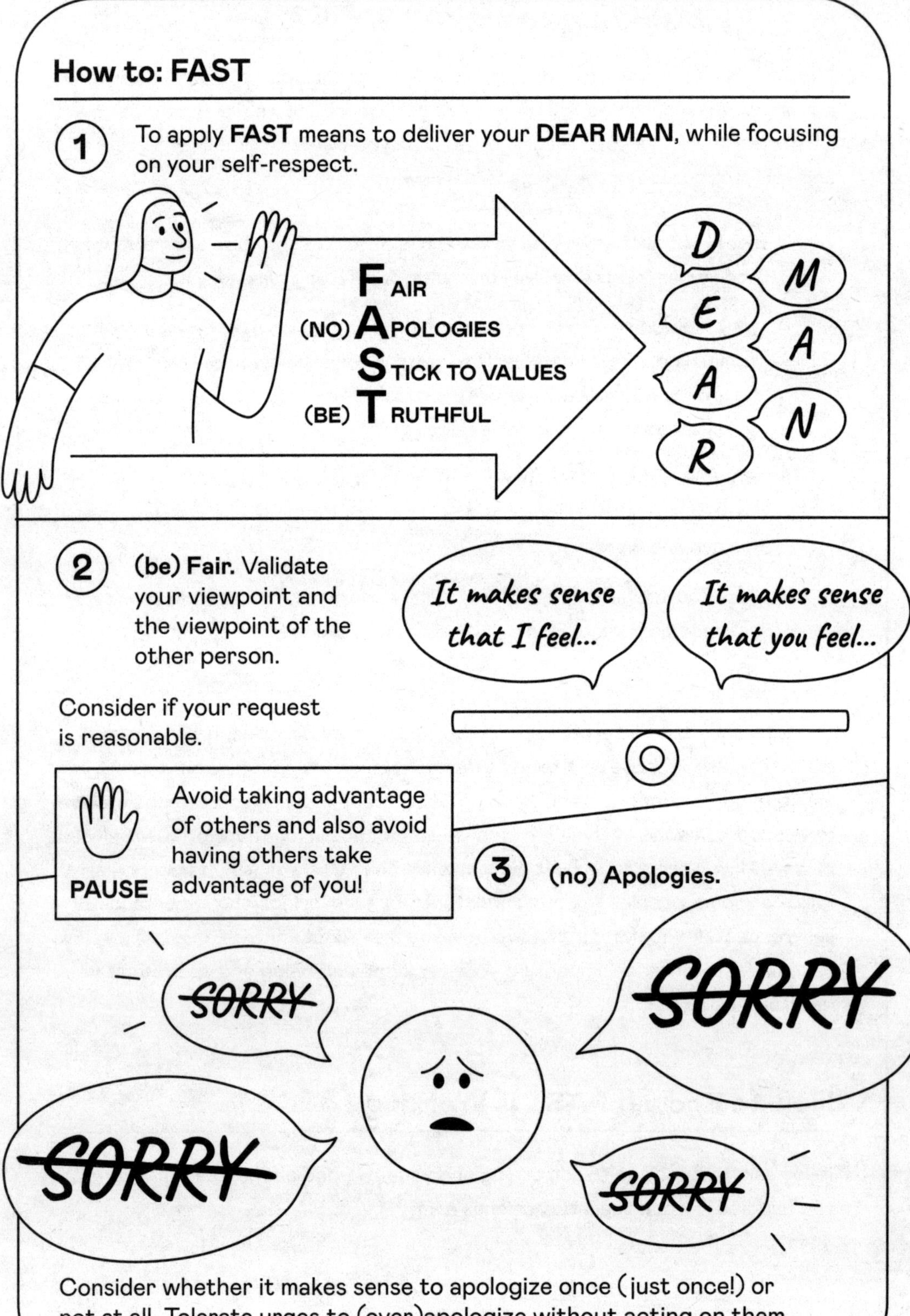
How to: FAST
1
To apply FAST means to deliver your DEAR MAN, while focusing on your self-respect.
FAIR
(NO) APOLOGIES
STICK TO VALUES
(BE) TRUTHFUL
D
E
A
R
M
A
N
2
(be) Fair. Validate your viewpoint and the viewpoint of the other person.
It makes sense that I feel...
It makes sense that you feel...
Consider if your request is reasonable.
PAUSE
Avoid taking advantage of others and also avoid having others take advantage of you!
3
(no) Apologies.
SORRY
SORRY
SORRY
SORRY
Consider whether it makes sense to apologize once (just once!) or not at all. Tolerate urges to (over)apologize without acting on them.

④ **Stick to values.** Consider how your request aligns with your values.

Why is asking for what I want or saying no important to me?

REQUEST

VALUES · VALUES · VALUES · VALUES · VAL

If your request is in line with your values, it's more than ok to ask for what you want.

Keeping your values in mind helps you stay firm and not waver.

⑤ **(be) Truthful.** If you notice urges to lie, practice your Describe skills and stick to the facts.

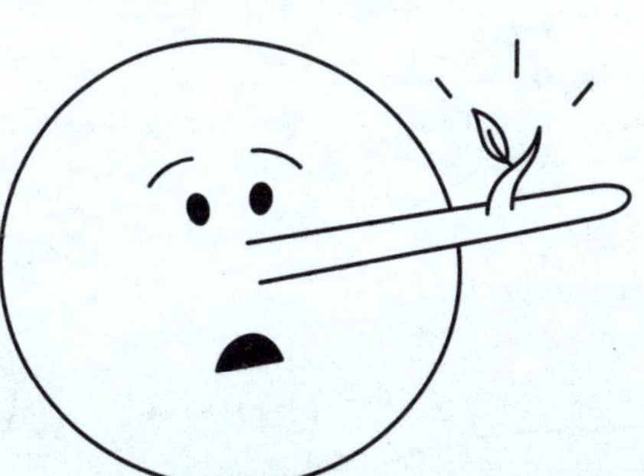

You can even make a note to yourself:

A lie may provide short-term relief and it will damage my long-term self-respect.

⑥ Ask someone to role-play with you so that you can practice all these elements in advance.

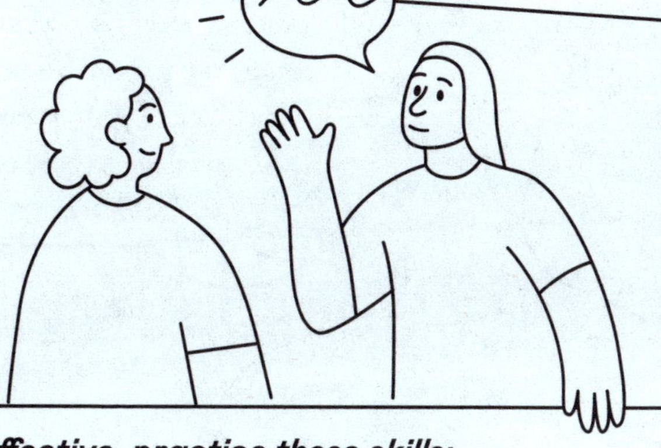

When FAST isn't effective, practice these skills:
SELF-SOOTHE · RADICAL ACCEPTANCE

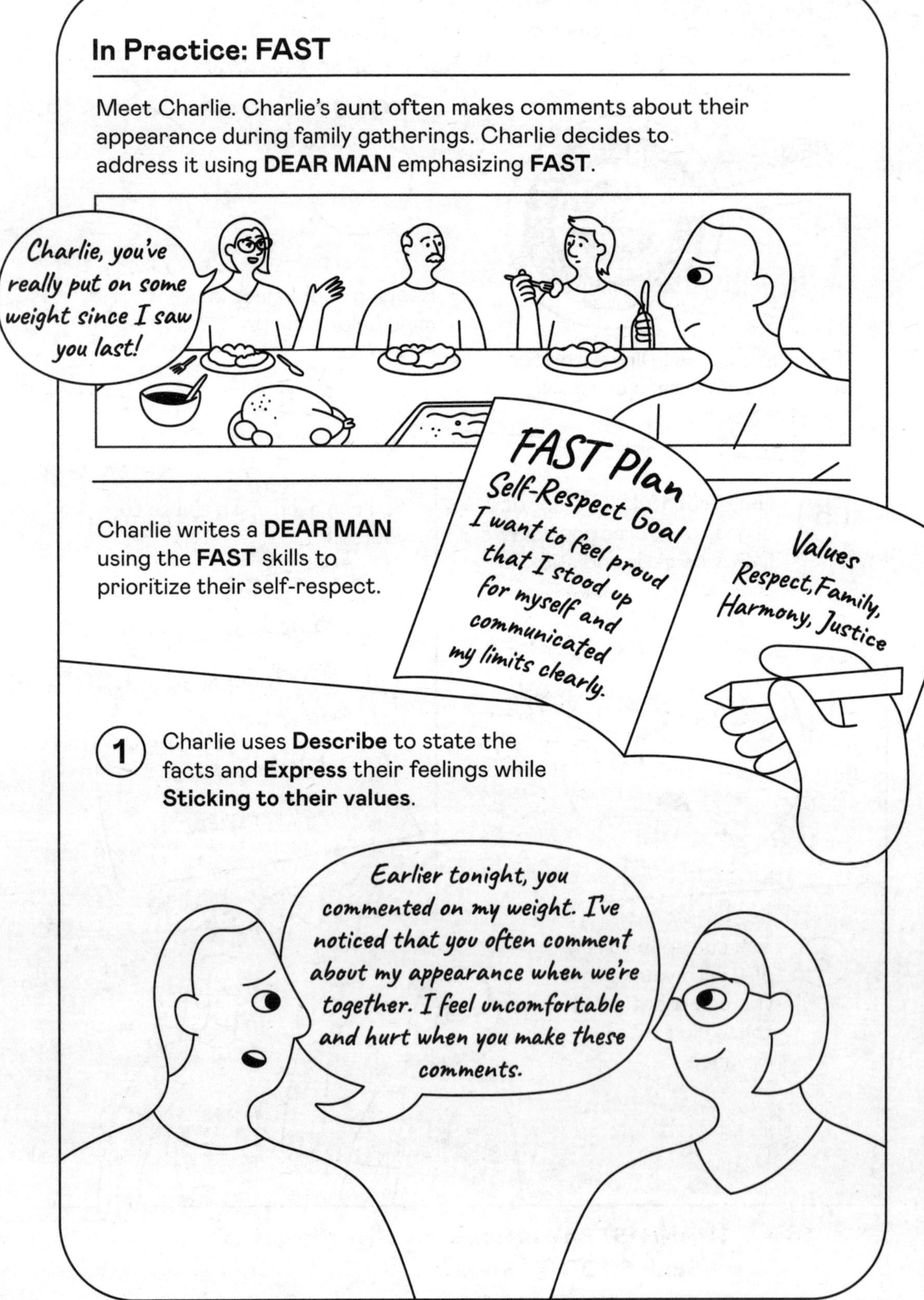
In Practice: FAST
Meet Charlie. Charlie's aunt often makes comments about their appearance during family gatherings. Charlie decides to address it using **DEAR MAN** emphasizing **FAST**.
Charlie, you've really put on some weight since I saw you last!
Charlie writes a **DEAR MAN** using the **FAST** skills to prioritize their self-respect.
FAST Plan
Self-Respect Goal
I want to feel proud that I stood up for myself and communicated my limits clearly.
Values
Respect, Family, Harmony, Justice
1 Charlie uses **Describe** to state the facts and **Express** their feelings while **Sticking to their values**.
Earlier tonight, you commented on my weight. I've noticed that you often comment about my appearance when we're together. I feel uncomfortable and hurt when you make these comments.

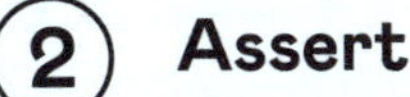

Assert

Charlie **Asserts** their request clearly.

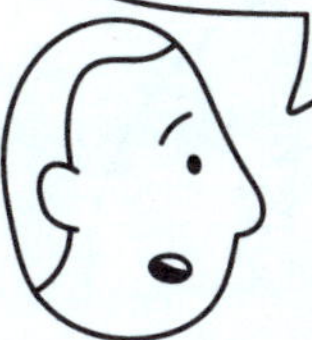
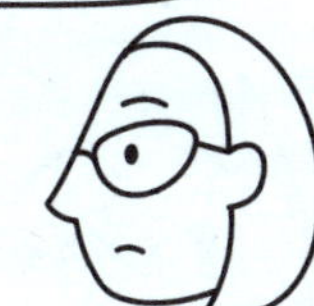

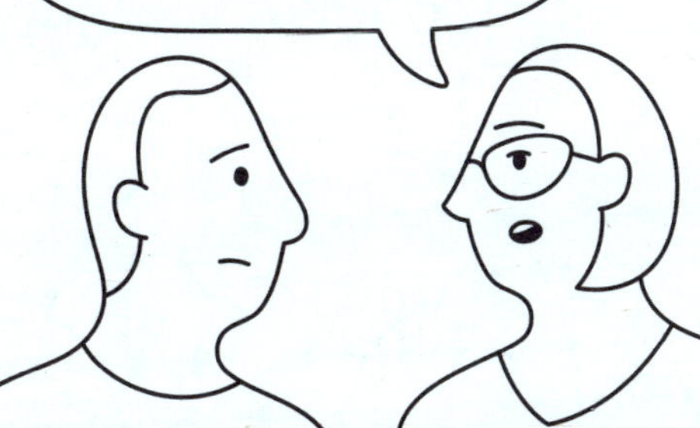

3 (no) Apologies and (be) Fair

Charlie practices **(no) Apologies**, **(be) Fair**, validating their aunt's perspective, and stays **Mindful** of their request.

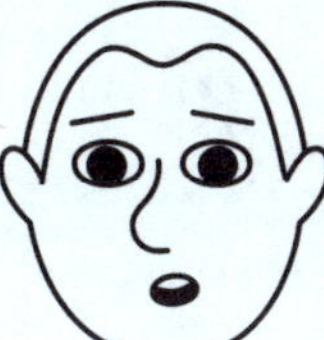

4 Reinforce

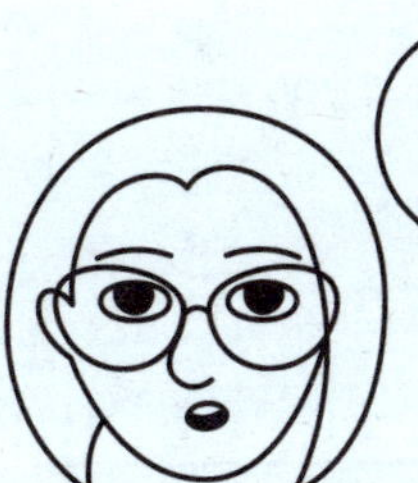

Charlie ends the conversation by **Reinforcing** their aunt's agreement.

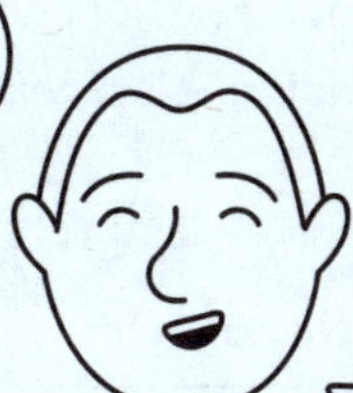

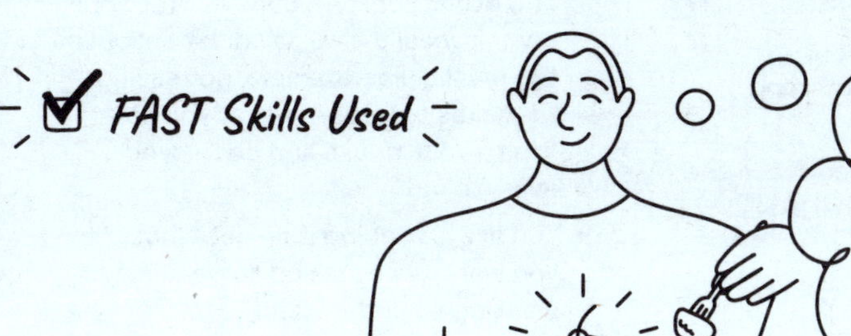

VALIDATION

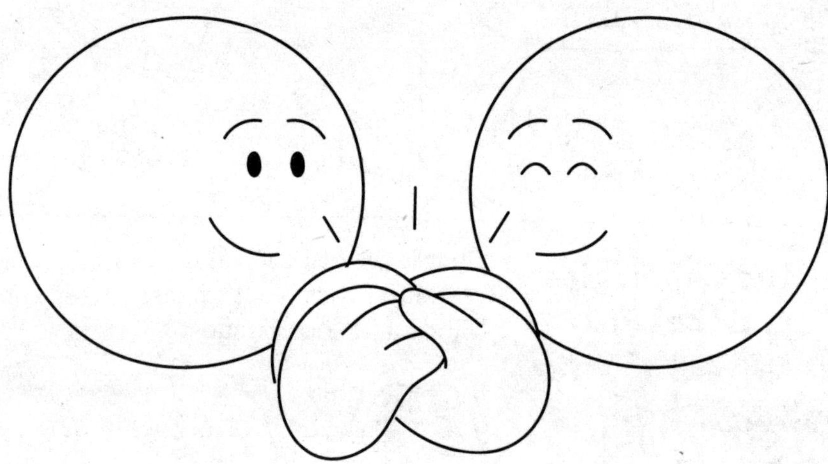

Why Use Validation?

Validation enhances your relationships by demonstrating that you are truly listening and understanding. It's a relationship superpower.

When to Use Validation

☑ **Use when:**

- You want to improve your relationships.
- You want to better understand another person.
- You want to be more effective in the use of other interpersonal skills.

☒ **Do NOT use when:**

- The other person's behavior (or your own) is *in*valid—we say don't validate the invalid. For example, not saying "it makes total sense that you set fire to your house and destroyed everything!"
- You are *just* doing it to get what you want (as opposed to genuinely wanting to understand).

VALIDATION is the act of acknowledging and affirming another person's perspective. Most of us know how good it feels to be validated; it allows us to feel understood and possibly closer to the person who is validating us. However, many of us never learned *how* to validate others or ourselves. The strategies in DBT offer specific methods for expressing validation in both verbal and nonverbal ways. Using validation regularly with others will increase the strength of our relationships and will also increase our effectiveness in moments of conflict or tension. When others feel understood by us, they are more likely to also see things from *our* perspective and may be more likely to agree to something we ask of them.

Validation means finding the kernel of truth in another person's perspective or behavior and communicating that we understand. It's saying "I get it" and meaning it. Even if we don't like what the other person is doing, or even if we disagree with their perspective, we can always find something to validate.

There are six specific ways to practice validation. You can use all of them in any conversation. Some of them can be done without specific words. Being fully present and fully participating in a conversation can be hugely validating to the other person. Other strategies involve verbally expressing understanding. Starting your sentences with "It makes sense that . . . " can be a good segue into validation. Like other skills in this book, initially it might feel awkward to use these strategies, especially if they don't come naturally to you. Keep at it.

How to Know If Validation Is Working

Validation is in the eye of the beholder—it's working if the other person feels validated. One way to determine this is to ask directly (*"Are you feeling like I get it?"*). If the person stays engaged in conversation and continues to open up, that might also be an indicator that Validation is working.

How to: Validation

There are six ways to validate.

1 Pay attention.

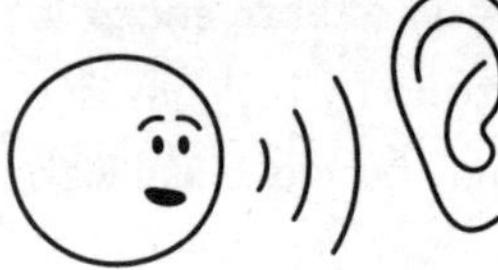

Be fully present while listening.

Make eye contact.

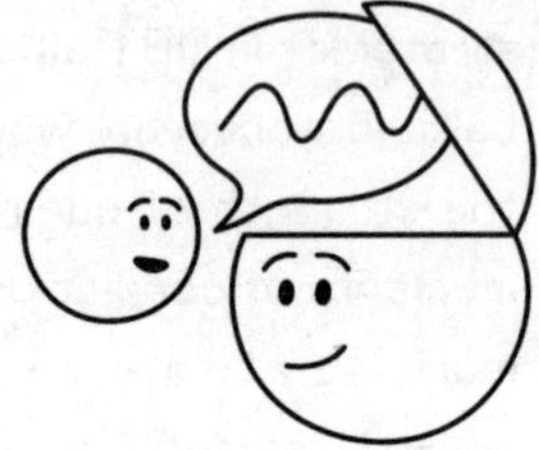

Take in what they're saying and doing.

PAUSE Don't be distracted or think about what you're going to say next.

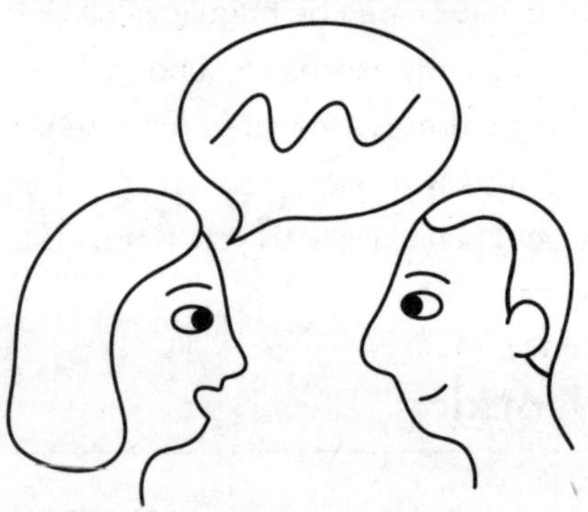

2 Reflect back.

Communicate that you understand what the other person is saying by summarizing and reflecting back to them.

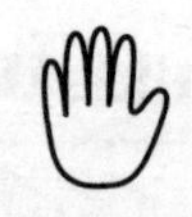

PAUSE Don't be a parrot. Instead, summarize back in your own words.

3 "Mindread."

Say out loud what the other person is not saying but may be thinking or feeling.

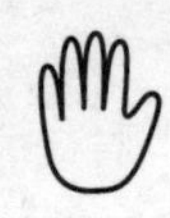

PAUSE Don't insist on your perspective. If they say you're wrong, believe them!

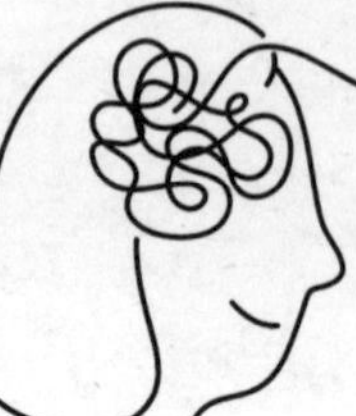

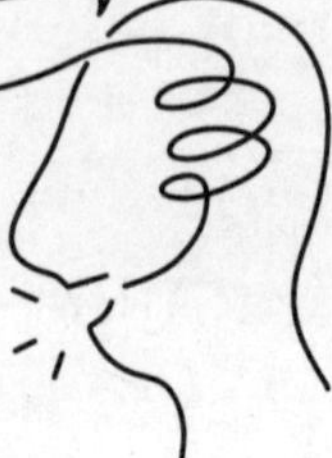

4 Express understanding.

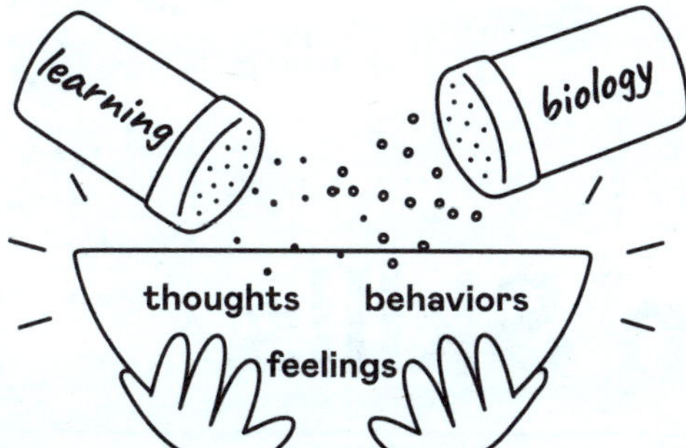

That makes so much sense given all you've been through.

Reflect how the person's thoughts, behaviors, or feelings make sense given their learning history or biology.

5 Acknowledge the valid.

Communicate what is understandable about the person's thoughts, behaviors, or feelings.

Highlight that their behavior makes sense and that most other people would feel similar in the same circumstance.

That makes total sense! Anyone would respond that way!

6 Show equality.

Also known as radical genuineness. Be completely yourself with the other person and treat them as a person of equal value to you.

PAUSE Don't talk down to them or condescend.

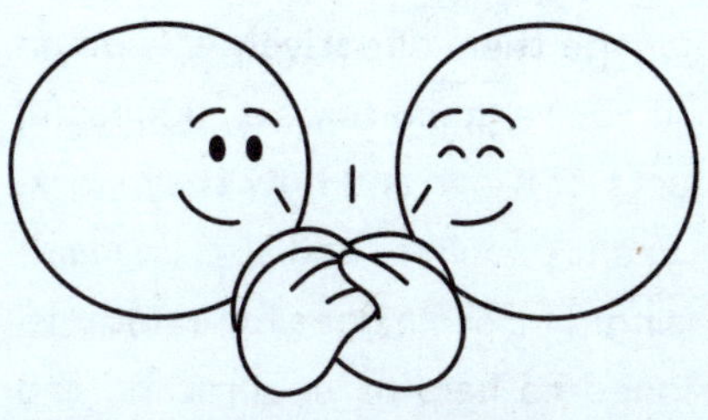

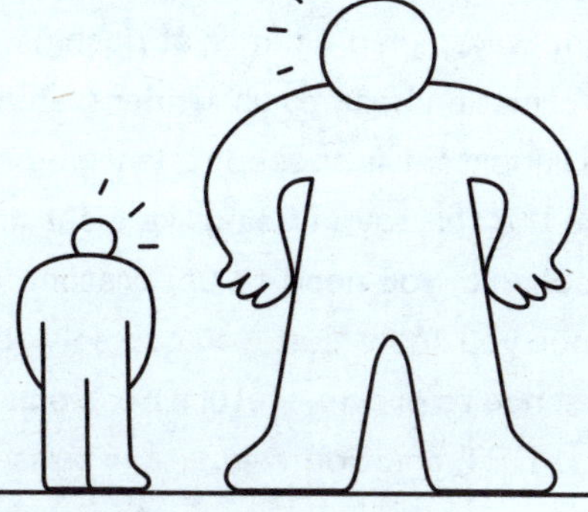

When Validation isn't effective, practice these skills:

CHAIN ANALYSIS (to assess what's really going on)

DEAR MAN · RADICAL ACCEPTANCE

Emotion Regulation Skills

AN OVERVIEW

To be human is to experience a range of emotions throughout our daily lives. We tend to like certain emotions—joy, interest, love—and want them to last as long as possible. We tend to dislike others—shame, sadness, fear—and want to avoid them or get them to end as quickly as we can. The truth is, all emotions are fleeting. Or at least they *can* be fleeting if we know how to respond to them.

In DBT, we first recognize that most of the time, our emotions are serving a very useful purpose: They keep us alive, motivate our behavior in important ways, keep us in relationships with others, and communicate important information back to us. Understanding which emotion(s) we're experiencing is an important first step to learning how to manage them effectively. We often use the analogy of being like a car mechanic: If you're going to be a successful mechanic, you need to understand all the parts of a car and how they work. Once you know that, you can solve a car's current problems and also do maintenance to prevent future problems from arising. The same goes for emotions. The DBT emotion regulation skills are designed to help us understand the parts of our emotions, more effectively manage emotions that cause us problems, and prevent future emotional problems. The skills include:

- Learning to understand our emotions (Model for Describing Emotions)
- Reducing our vulnerability to Emotion Mind (PLEASE skills)
- Creating more positive emotional experiences (ABC skills)
- Learning how to change emotions that we don't want (Check the Facts, Opposite Action, Problem Solving)
- Incorporating mindfulness to ride the wave of our emotions when we have them (Mindfulness of Current Emotions)

As you'll soon realize, if you didn't know this already, emotions are complex full-body experiences that include physical sensations, thoughts, urges, and behaviors. They are typically comprised of several parts or reactions all happening at once. Given everything that occurs when we experience emotions, it's no wonder that we often struggle to manage them. These skills provide a rich array of possible responses to emotional experiences. With practice, they will lead you to feel less stuck and more in control.

MODEL FOR DESCRIBING EMOTIONS

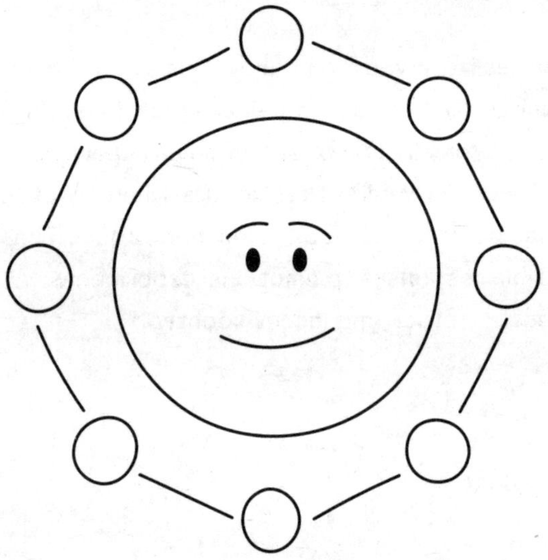

Why Use Model for Describing Emotions?

This skill helps us understand why we feel a certain way, as well as understand what can and can't be changed about how we feel.

When to Use Model for Describing Emotions

☑ **Use when:**

You are feeling something but aren't sure what. The Model is almost always helpful for getting us to accurately describe what we're feeling. The Model is often a precursor to another skill designed to help you change or accept your emotions.

☒ **Do NOT use when:**

- You already have a pretty good idea of what you're feeling.
- You are in a crisis and need to act immediately.

THE MODEL FOR DESCRIBING EMOTIONS ("the Model") explains what an emotion actually is—all the parts that comprise an emotion and lead us to "feel" a certain way. The Model has a number of components (see pages 78–79) and is divided into three sections: antecedents, the emotion experience, and consequences. You can modify some of these elements, but not all of them. This is important! We often try to talk ourselves out of feeling something when, in fact, we don't have control over it.

Emotion science is a huge field and it could take several books to describe this fully. The Model provides a simple overview to get you started on understanding your emotions more clearly.

Antecedents are the components that come before, and lead to, the experience of the emotion.

- The *prompting event* is an event or situation that occurs right before the emotion starts, like the cue that sets off the emotion in that moment. Prompting events can be external, like someone saying something rude to you, or internal, like a nightmare.
- *Vulnerability factors* refer to conditions or events that make us more vulnerable to the prompting event in that given moment. Maybe some days you can quickly brush off someone being rude, but other days, you ruminate on it for hours. That's likely because vulnerability factors are playing a role. Vulnerability factors include things like being tired, hungry, in physical pain, or stressed.
- *Interpretations* refer to our thoughts about the prompting event. Often what sets off our emotion is our interpretation of an event, rather than the event itself. For example, having the thought "I have a terminal illness" in response to a headache arising will likely lead to fear and anxiety, as opposed to having the thought "here's another unpleasant headache that I have to experience before it goes away with some pain relievers," which will likely not elicit fear or anxiety.

Important note about antecedents: We can change our experience of an emotion by changing any of these pieces. Many of the skills in this book teach us how to do exactly that (for example, PLEASE, page 84; Check the Facts, page 92; Problem Solving, page 100).

The emotion experience includes the elements that comprise our experience of an emotion. In the illustration (page 79), the column on the left lists elements that we cannot directly change or control: biological changes, action urges, and body sensations.

- *Biological changes* include brain changes, neural firings, and nervous system changes that impact things like neurochemistry, heart rate, hormone levels, perspiration, and other autonomic changes.
- *Body sensations* are typically what we experience when we say we "feel" sad, angry, or ashamed. For example, sadness often goes along with sensations of low energy and heaviness in limbs and chest.
- *Action urges* are what we *feel* like doing. For example, the phrase "fight, flight, or freeze" refers to action urges that go along with the experience of fear. All emotions have urges that occur with them. We can't change the urges we feel but we can choose to act on them or not.

The column on the right lists elements that we generally have more control over: face and body language, words, and actions.

- *Face and body language* refers to how our face and body look and, importantly, how they convey what we are feeling. What do your face and body look like when you are sad? How does this differ from what your face and body look like when you are angry?
- *Words* are what we say.
- *Actions* are what we do, or what behavior we engage in.

Important note about the emotion experience: Changing any part of the system can have an effect on the whole experience, but it's important to recognize that we can't control all of the pieces.

Consequences are the components that follow an emotional experience.

- *Emotional awareness* refers to labeling our emotional experience. Naming our experience as "shame," "anger," or "joy," for example, can increase our mindful experience of our emotions and lead us to better deploy other skills that may help us in the moment.

- *Aftereffects* are what we experience after an intense emotion that can often make us vulnerable to a new emotional experience (or the same emotional experience again). Intense emotions often have an effect on thoughts, memory, physical functioning, and ability to think clearly. For example, after an intense feeling of fear when you think your life is in danger, you might feel shaky, on edge, and have difficulty concentrating even after the threat is gone. And this might make you on the lookout for other threatening cues that indicate danger and prompt more fear.
- *Secondary emotions* are emotions that may be prompted by an initial emotional experience. Have you ever noticed, for example, that when you feel intense shame, you are quick to lash out in anger at someone else? That anger is considered a secondary emotion to shame. It's important to distinguish primary and secondary emotions because often we try to change our emotional experiences by targeting the secondary emotion when it would be more effective to work on the primary one.

Important note about consequences: Consequences play a critical role in how long an emotional experience seems to last for us. Emotions themselves are very short-lived, often lasting seconds or minutes. Yet, our experience of emotions is that they frequently last much longer than this. That's likely because we do things when we experience emotions that keep them around. A common refrain in DBT is that "emotions love themselves." If we learn to change how we respond to emotions, we can decrease the amount of time we spend in emotional suffering.

How to Know If Model for Describing Emotions Is Working

The outcome of going through the Model for Describing Emotions is to have better clarity about your emotional experience. In and of itself, the Model doesn't lead to change. However, you may find that being able to label your emotions in a nonjudgmental way improves your capacity to manage how you're feeling more effectively.

Model of Emotions

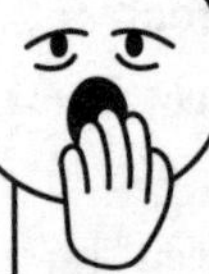

VULNERABILITY FACTORS

Vulnerability factors are the conditions that make you more sensitive to the **prompting event**.

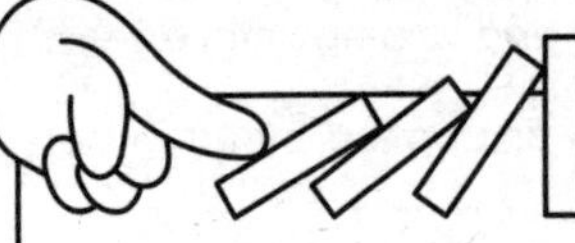

PROMPTING EVENT

The **prompting event** is the situation that sparks an **emotion**.

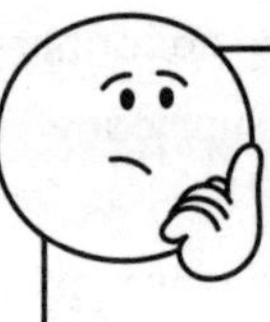

INTERPRETATIONS

Interpretations are the thoughts we have about the **prompting event**.

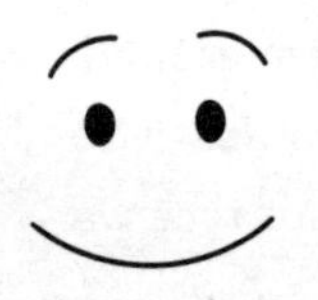

EMOTION

An **emotion** is a response elicited by the **prompting event** or the **interpretation** of the **event**. It has several elements—see next page. ★

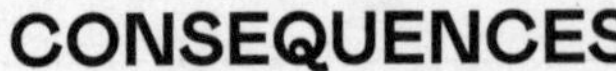

CONSEQUENCES

The consequences **of an emotion** may include recognizing the emotion, secondary emotions, and aftereffects like other thoughts and sensations.

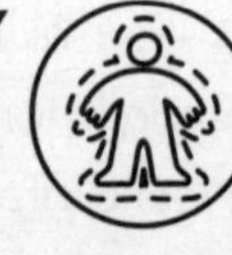

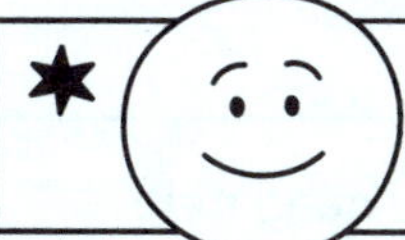

ELEMENTS OF AN EMOTION

INTERNAL

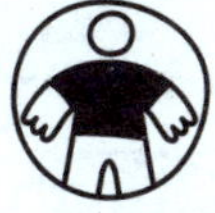

EXTERNAL

BIOLOGICAL CHANGES include shifts in heart rate, breathing, neurochemistry, and hormone levels.

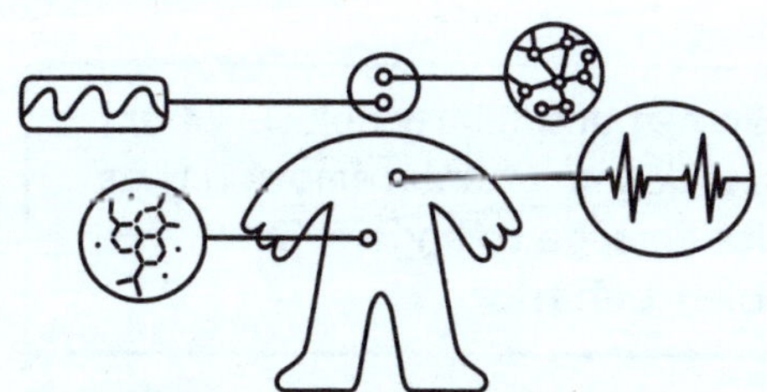

FACE AND BODY LANGUAGE are how we show and communicate our emotions.

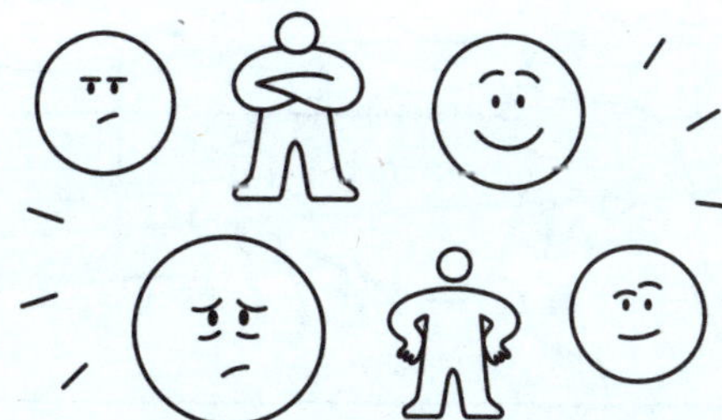

BODY SENSATIONS are the physical feelings tied to emotions, like the heaviness we may feel when sad.

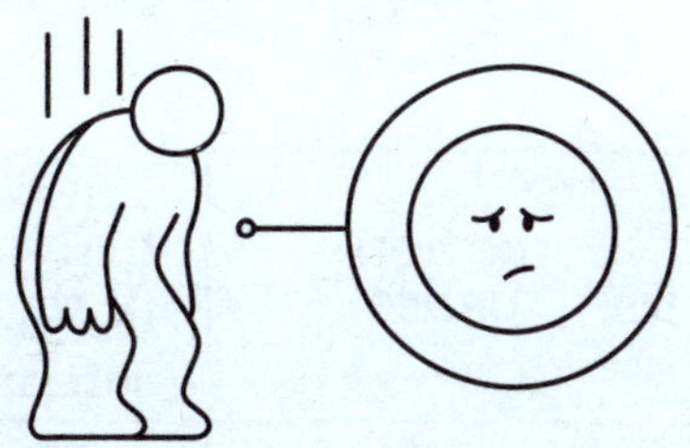

WORDS are what we say when we have an emotion.

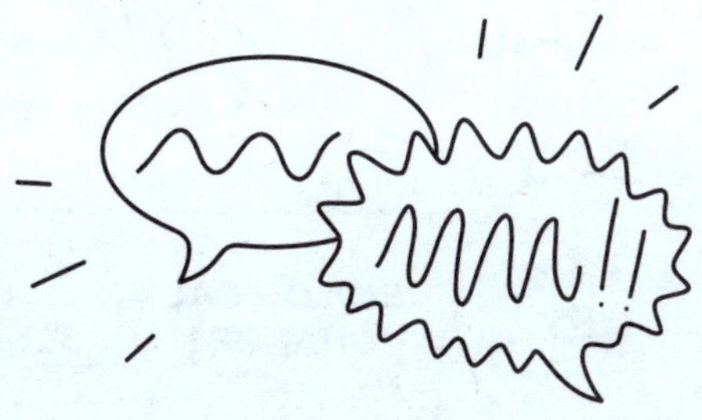

ACTION URGES are responses generated by the brain to prepare the body for action.

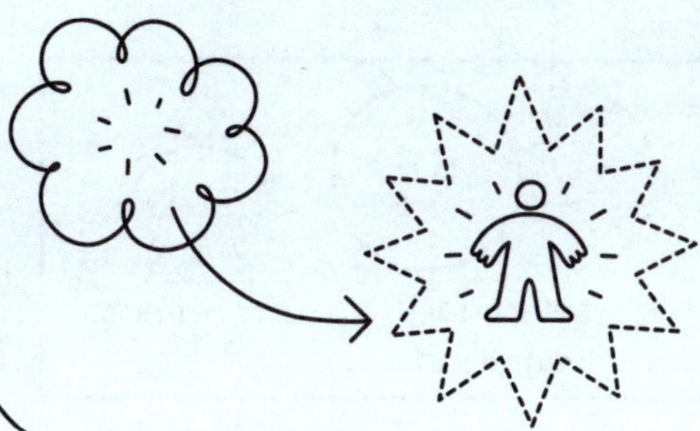

ACTIONS are what we do when we experience an emotion.

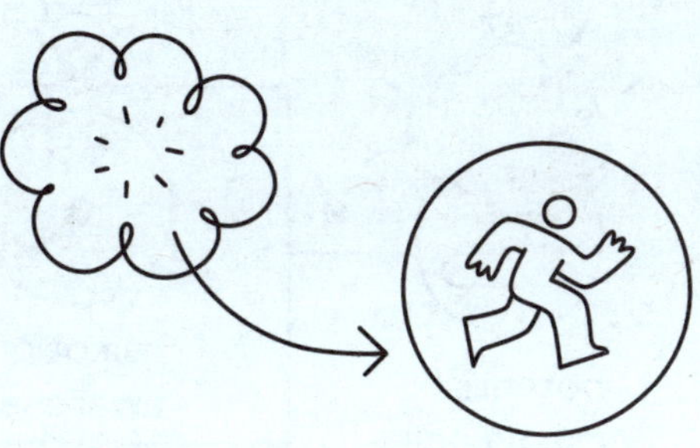

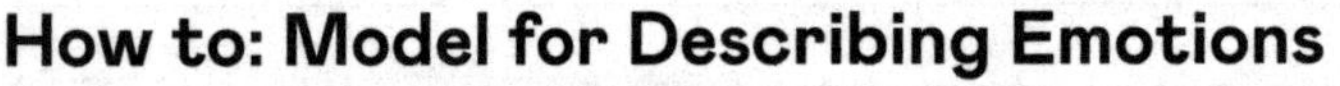

How to: Model for Describing Emotions

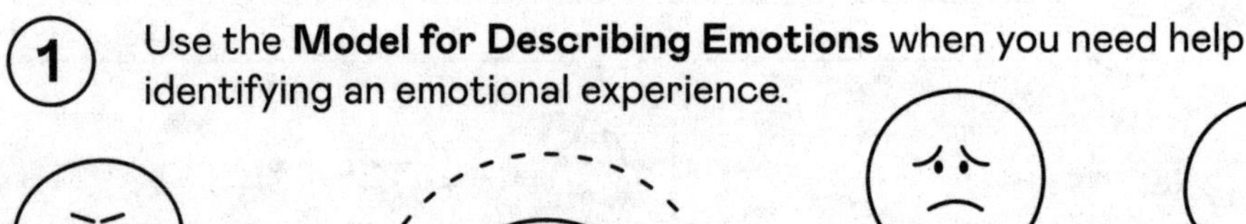

1. Use the **Model for Describing Emotions** when you need help identifying an emotional experience.

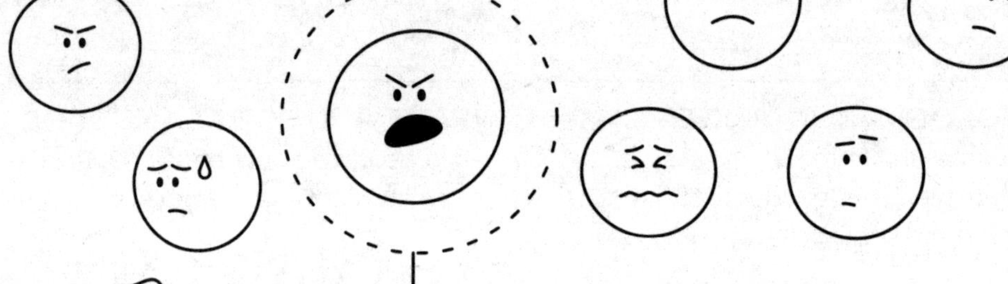

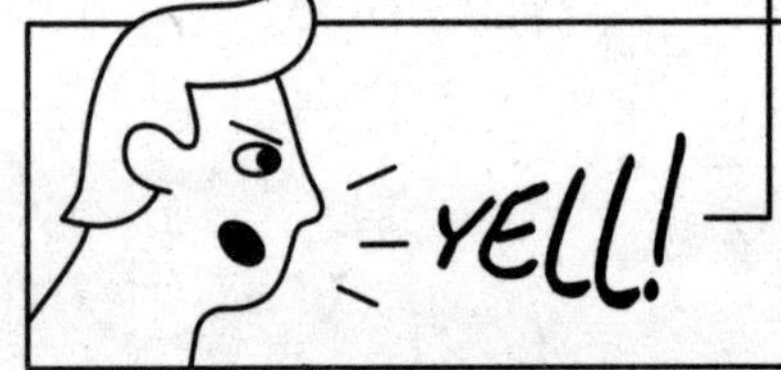

It can be particularly helpful when you notice an intense emotion that elicits an urge to engage in a problem behavior.

2. Refer to the **Model of Emotions** diagram shown earlier. Pick any of the elements in the diagram to begin.

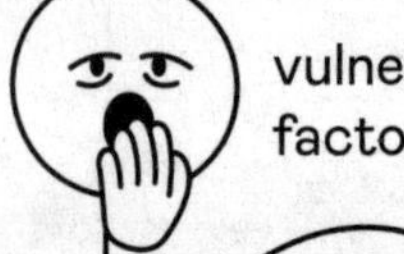

vulnerability factors

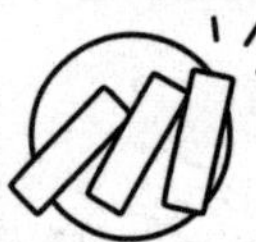

prompting event

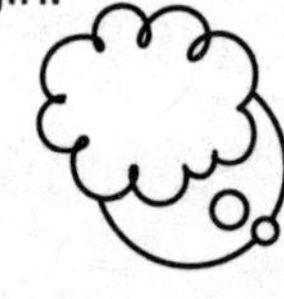

interpretation

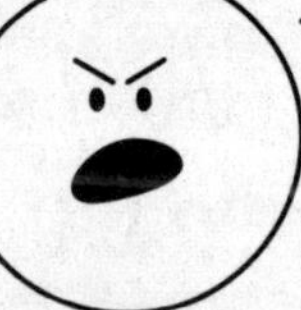

emotion

BIOLOGICAL CHANGES

BODY SENSATIONS

ACTION URGES

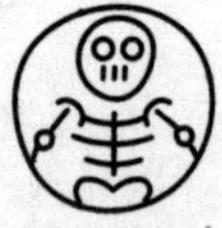

internal

FACE AND BODY LANGUAGE

WORDS

ACTIONS

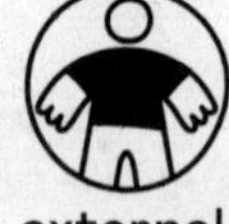

external

potential consequences

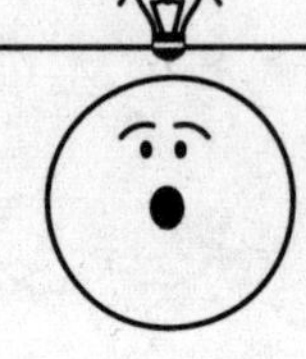

emotion awareness

secondary emotion

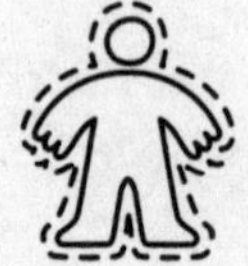

aftereffects

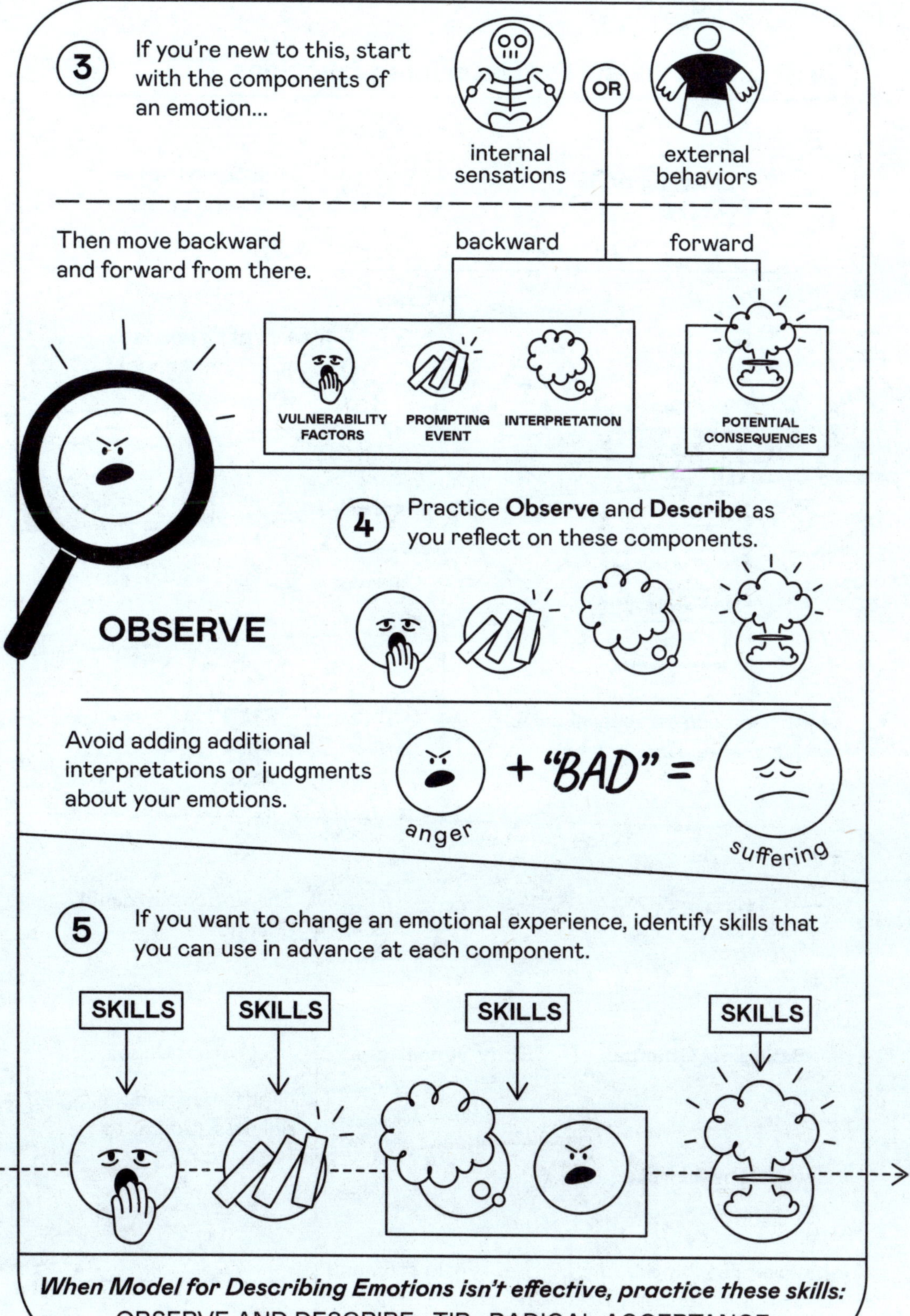

When Model for Describing Emotions isn't effective, practice these skills:

OBSERVE AND DESCRIBE · TIP · RADICAL ACCEPTANCE

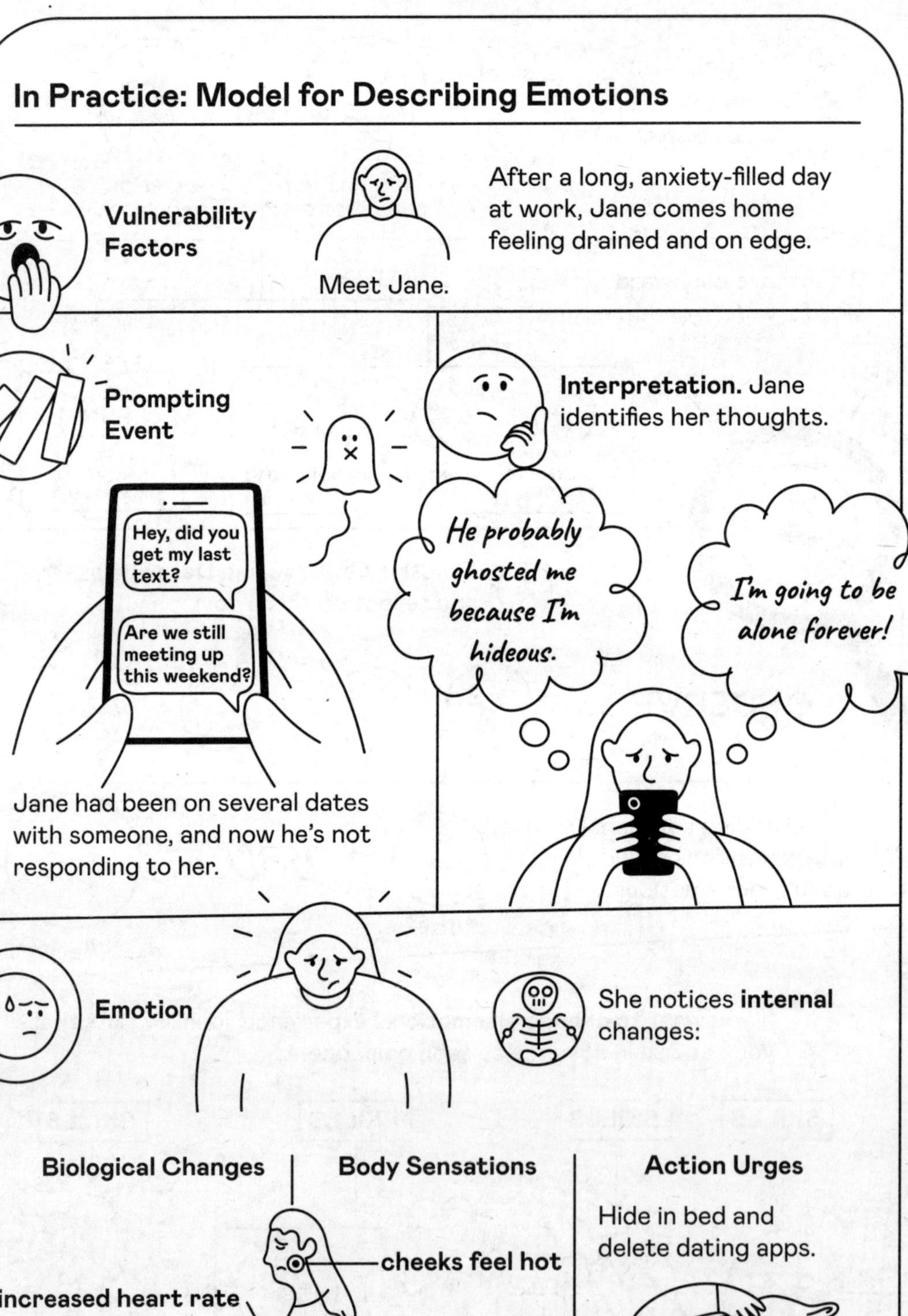
In Practice: Model for Describing Emotions
Vulnerability Factors
Meet Jane.
After a long, anxiety-filled day at work, Jane comes home feeling drained and on edge.
Prompting Event
Hey, did you get my last text?
Are we still meeting up this weekend?
Jane had been on several dates with someone, and now he's not responding to her.
Interpretation. Jane identifies her thoughts.
He probably ghosted me because I'm hideous.
I'm going to be alone forever!
Emotion
She notices internal changes:
Biological Changes
Body Sensations
cheeks feel hot
increased heart rate
shallow breathing
pit in stomach
Action Urges
Hide in bed and delete dating apps.

She observes **external** changes:

Face and Body Language

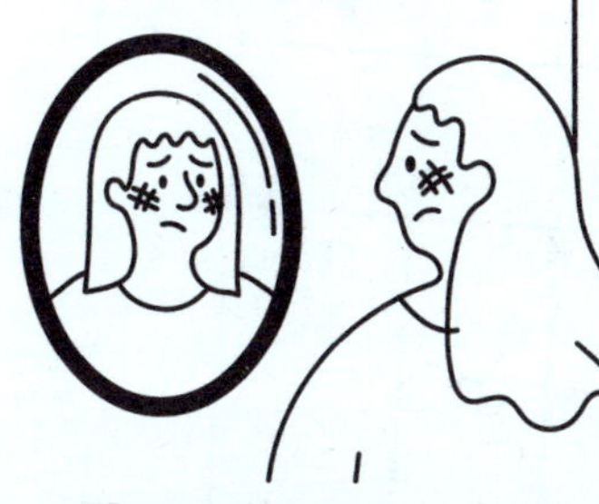

Flushed cheeks.
Shoulders slumped.
Eyes downcast.

Words

I'm such a loser.

Actions

She withdraws from her roommate, and doom scrolls to escape.

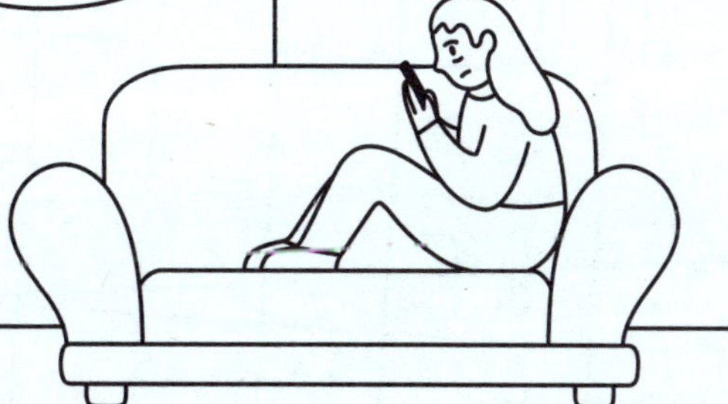

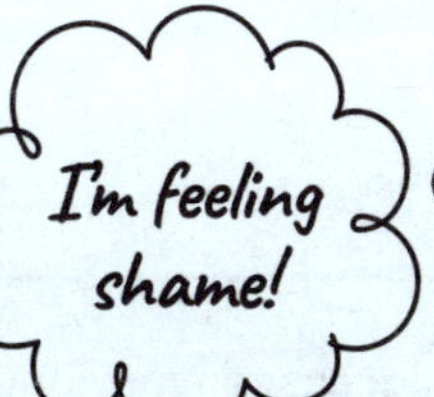

Consequences. Jane notices that this emotional experience is sticking around and getting more intense.

Emotion Awareness

I'm feeling shame!

Secondary Emotions

Jane starts to feel anger at herself and the guy.

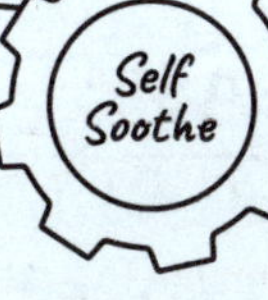

Aftereffects

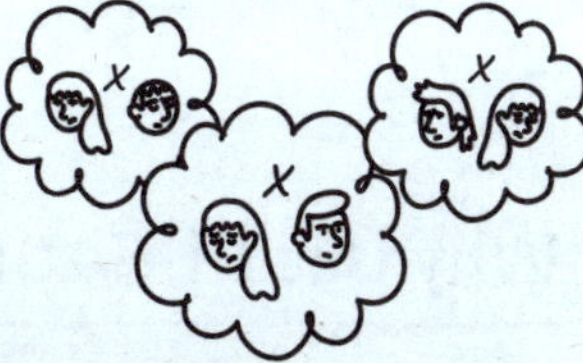

Jane thinks about all her other "failed" relationships.

By using the **Model for Describing Emotions**, Jane understands why shame and anger make sense.

Now she can find skills to help her manage this experience more effectively.

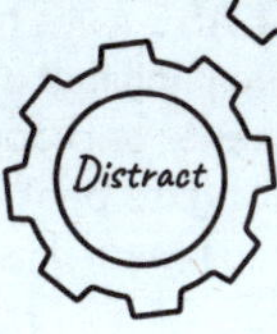

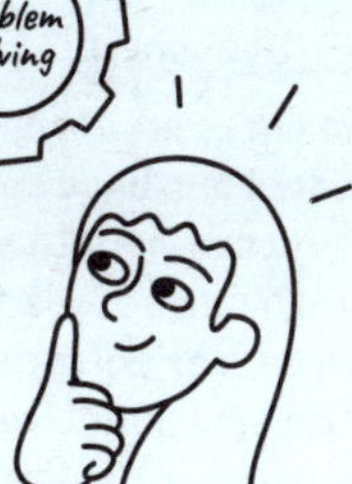

PLEASE

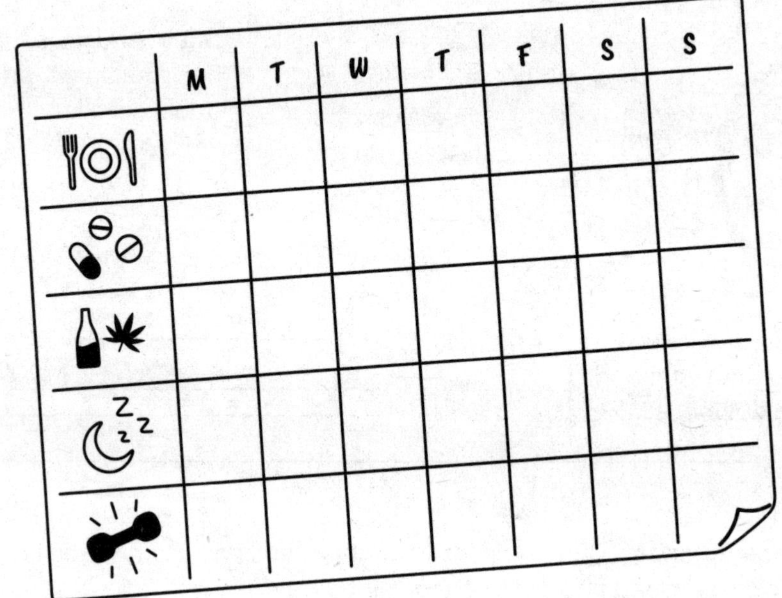

Why Use PLEASE?

PLEASE makes us less vulnerable to Emotion Mind and increases emotional resilience.

When to Use PLEASE

☑ **Use when:**

Ideally, every day! PLEASE skills help us feel our best and help mitigate the effects of negative events and conflicts. When our body is feeling its best, we are better equipped to handle life's problems effectively.

☒ **Do NOT use when:**

Responding to an immediate crisis. Because PLEASE refers to skills that require attention on a regular basis, they are usually not great for responding to an immediate crisis.

PLEASE is a (clunky) acronym used to describe what we can do to reduce our vulnerability to Emotion Mind. Most of us are aware that we feel more poorly when we are ill, eat too much or too little, use drugs and alcohol, sleep too much or too little, and lack exercise. We can't fully control negative events in our lives. However, we can control how vulnerable we may be to those negative events by taking care of our body. PLEASE skills are to be used daily to have their greatest effect. The skills include:

PL (treating) Physical iLlness: Take steps to prevent illness and take adequate care of yourself when you are sick, like having regular checkups, taking medications as prescribed, and resting when ill.

E (balanced) Eating: Make sure your daily consumption is good for you: not too much, not too little, lots of protein and vegetables, fewer sugars and fats. There's a lot of individual variability here; it will take some trial and error to figure out what balanced eating means for you. If you're aware that certain foods or eating at certain times of day make you more vulnerable to Emotion Mind, then work on avoiding those.

A Avoid mood-altering drugs and alcohol: For most people, using drugs and alcohol increases vulnerability to Emotion Mind and avoiding substances altogether is beneficial. If you're going to use substances, then do it mindfully and with awareness of how it affects you in both the short and the long term.

S (balanced) Sleep: Make sure you're getting the right amount of sleep for you. Most adults need 7–9 hours per night to feel their best. Take steps to increase your chances of getting more restorative sleep.

E Exercise: Aim to do some form of exercise every day for at least 20 minutes. If you are new to exercise, start small and build slowly over time. Do some activity that gets your heart rate up.

How to Know If PLEASE Is Working

You may notice PLEASE working when you observe fewer mood swings, a more consistent energy level, and easier access to Wise Mind when you're in stressful situations. Essentially, your emotional baseline becomes steadier, and your physical health supports your emotional well-being.

How to: PLEASE

1. Start by taking stock of each **PLEASE** skill. It might be helpful for you to make a **PLEASE** chart to keep track of food intake, medications, alcohol/drug consumption, sleep and wake time, and exercise.

	M	T	W	T	F	S	S
MEALS							
MEDICATIONS							
ALCOHOL/ DRUGS							
WAKE/ SLEEP							
EXERCISE							

2. **PL:** For treating physical illness, go to the doctor regularly and take medications as prescribed.

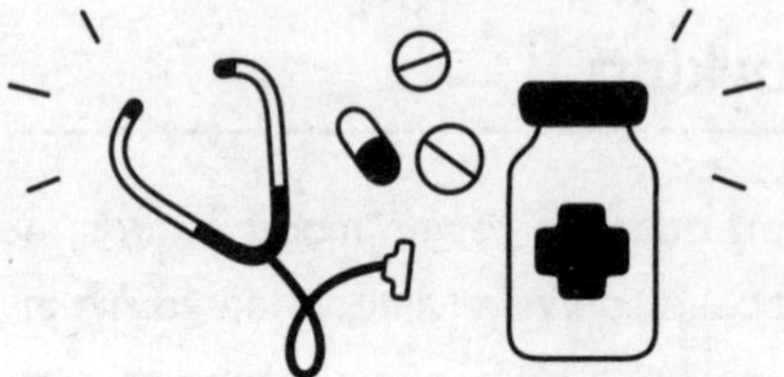

Slow down when you're sick and give yourself time to recover from illness or injury.

3. 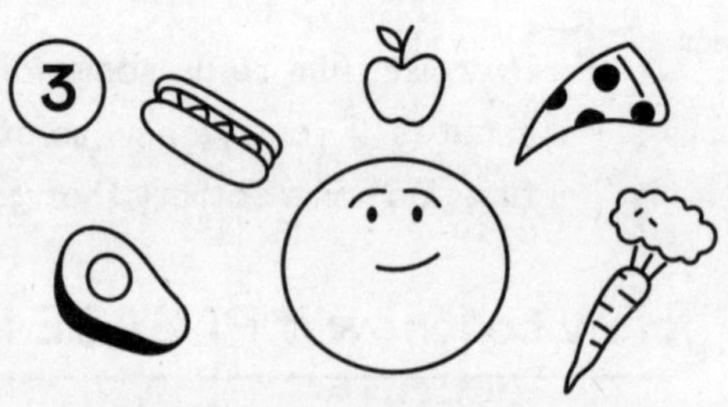

E: Take action to achieve more balanced eating. For example, plan meals ahead, avoid foods that make you feel overly emotional, or introduce foods that you have been restricting.

4 **A:** Use the **Pros/Cons** skill to understand how substances impact your mood and actions in the short and the long term.

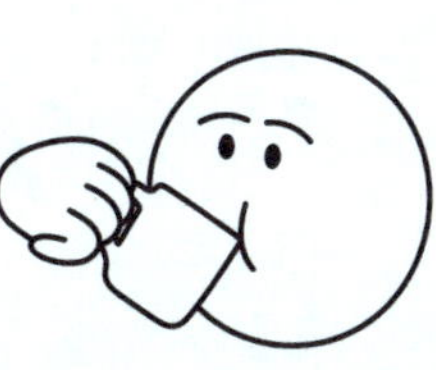
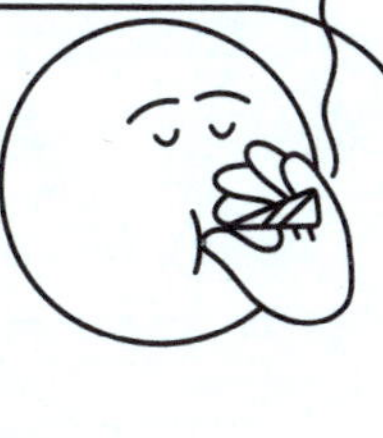

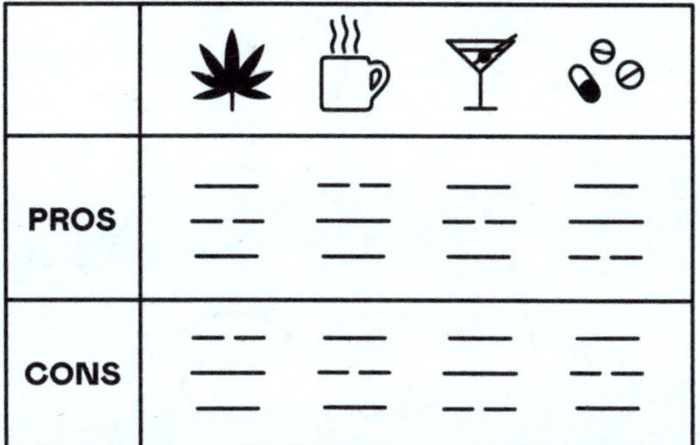

Include alcohol, drugs, cannabis products, caffeine, and over-the-counter medications.

Determine whether you want to cut back on your use of these substances or quit them altogether.

5 **S:** For balanced sleep, ask yourself if you're getting the right amount of sleep for you and your body.

Using a sleep tracker or journal, document your sleep schedule.

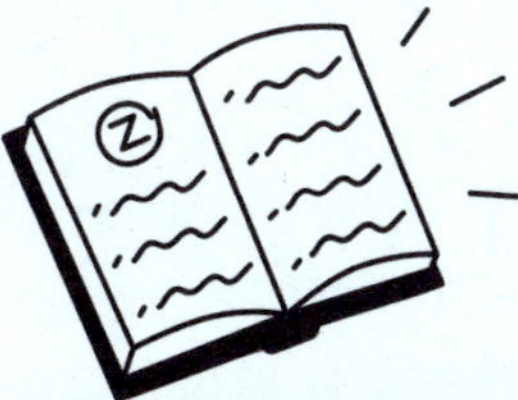

Seek out **cognitive-behavioral therapy for insomnia (CBT-I)** if you experience persistent sleep problems.

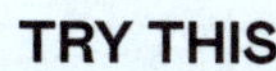

TRY THIS

To achieve more balanced sleep, try going to bed and waking up at the same times every day. Sleep in a cool, dark room. Only use your bed for sleep and romance.

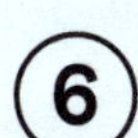

6 **E:** Pick a physical activity you enjoy, that gets your heart rate up, and that you can do regularly. Aim for at least 20 minutes of exercise a day. Any movement is good, whether it's brisk walking, dancing, or even cleaning.

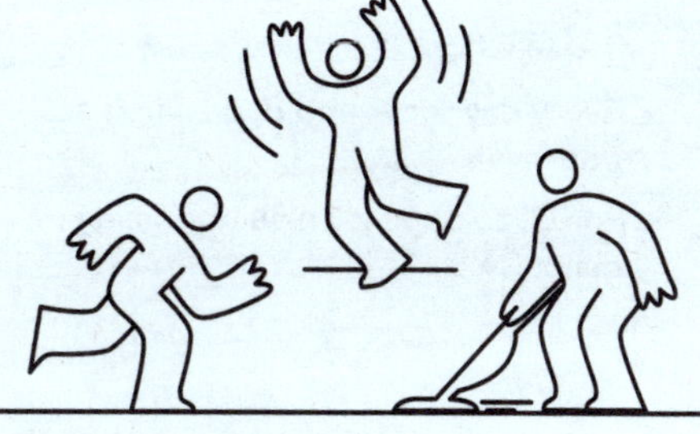

When PLEASE isn't effective, practice these skills:

DISTRACT · IMPROVE · TIP

ABC

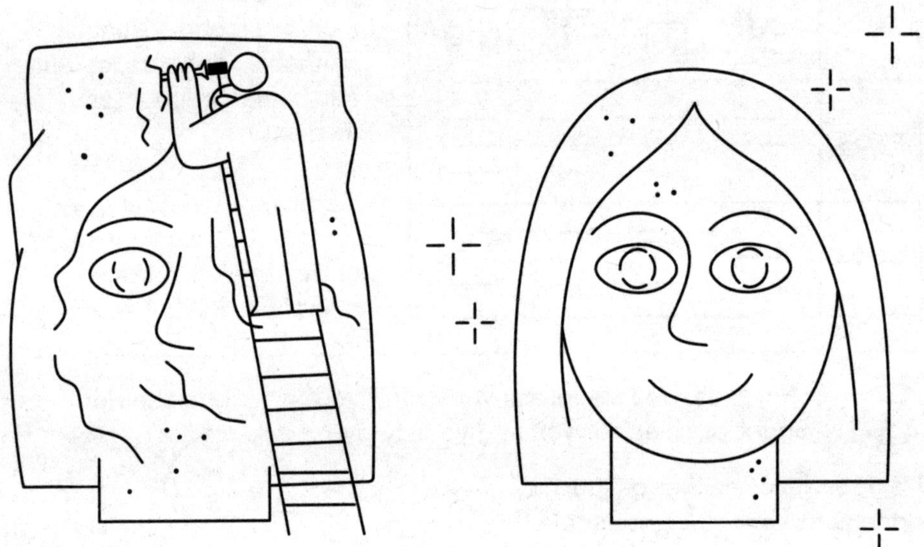

Why Use ABC?

ABC increases positive emotions and, by doing so, further reduces vulnerability to Emotion Mind.

When to Use ABC

☑ **Use when:**

- Every day for A and B, as much as possible!
- For C, to cope with an upcoming difficulty.

☒ **Do NOT use when:**

You're trying to avoid a different challenging task. That is, deciding to practice accumulating positives and going to the movies when you have an immediate school or work deadline is likely not effective. However, taking a 5-minute break to do something enjoyable is likely effective.

THE ABC skills are three skills designed to help reduce vulnerability to Emotion Mind, similar to PLEASE, by adding more positive experiences into your life. Together, these skills are like putting pennies in an emotional piggy bank: The more you have in your piggy bank, the less effect a withdrawal (unpleasant emotion experience or stressor) will have on you.

- A Accumulate positives: Add both short-term and long-term positives to your life. A short-term positive is doing something that immediately gives you a sense of pleasure or joy. It does not have to be big! A long-term positive is doing something that helps you get closer to a long-term goal. This often means doing something that you don't like (for example, studying for an exam) but is necessary for long-term success and pleasure.
- B Build mastery: Do something that gives you a sense of accomplishment and/or makes you feel competent. This may be something that you have been avoiding. Often this skill is referred to as an antidote to depression because it increases feelings of self-efficacy and self-worth.
- C Cope ahead: This skill refers to imagining an upcoming difficult situation or stressor and rehearsing yourself coping with it effectively. Mental practice will make a successful navigation of this experience more likely.

How to Know If ABC Is Working

ABC is working when you experience more moments of joy, pleasure, and accomplishment in your life. The goal is not to experience these constantly—that's impossible! Rather, the goal is to have daily experiences, which, like the PLEASE skills, will promote your overall sense of well-being. You may also notice that you're less likely to avoid doing difficult things the more you practice the ABC skills.

How to: ABC

Accumulate positives (short term).

Do something every day that gives you a sense of pleasure. It can be for just 5 minutes. Include activities that don't cost a lot (or any) money so that they're easier to sustain.

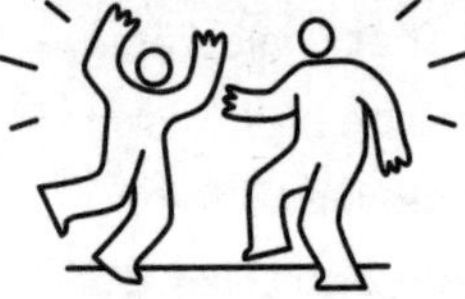

dance to your favorite song

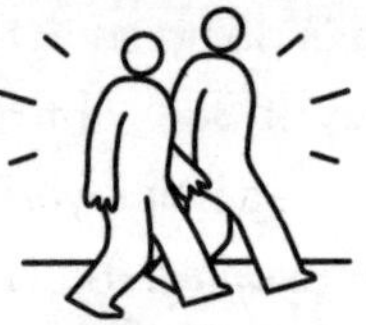

go for a walk with a friend

read an engaging book

go see art at a museum

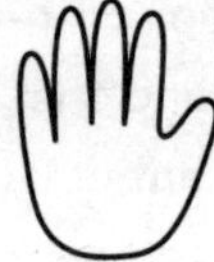

PAUSE

Fully **participate** in these activities—let go of worries and distractions. Don't let thoughts that you don't deserve it get in the way of this skill!

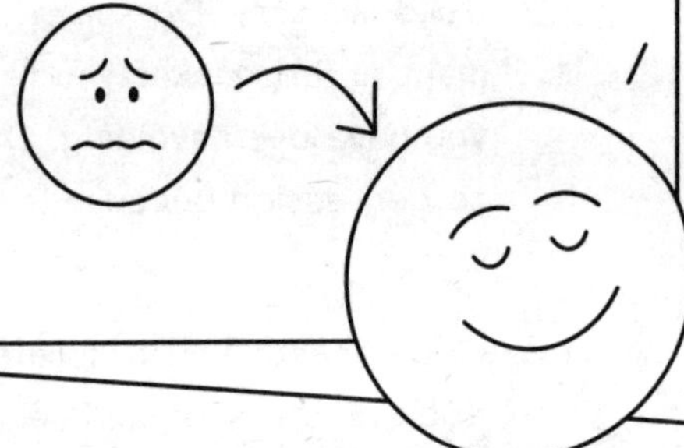

2 Accumulate positives (long term).

Do something every day that helps you get closer to a long-term goal.

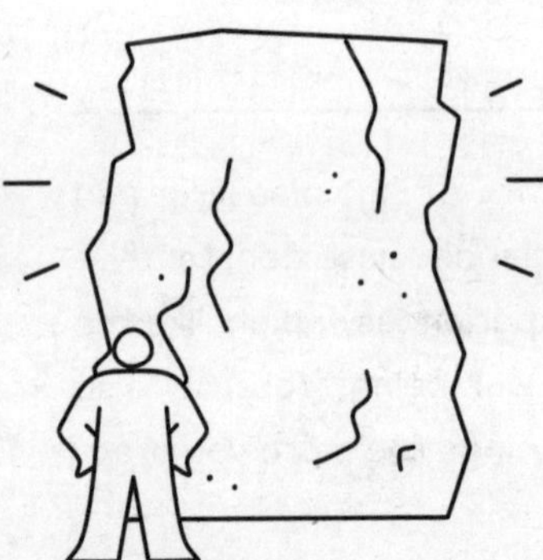

Recognize that achieving a long-term goal is actually a series of very small steps. Take the next step, no matter how small.

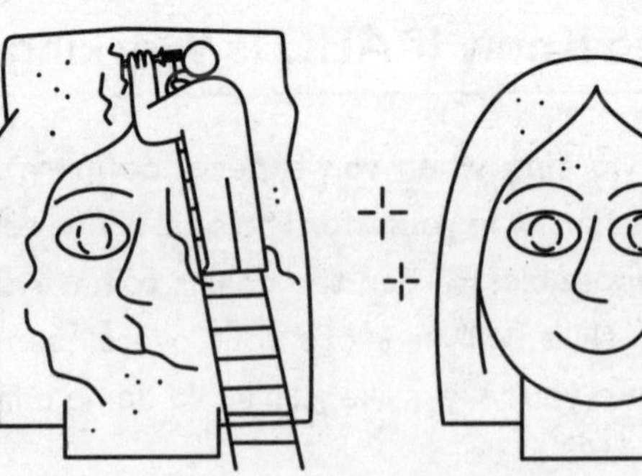

Do it mindfully (with full awareness) and reward yourself after you've done it.

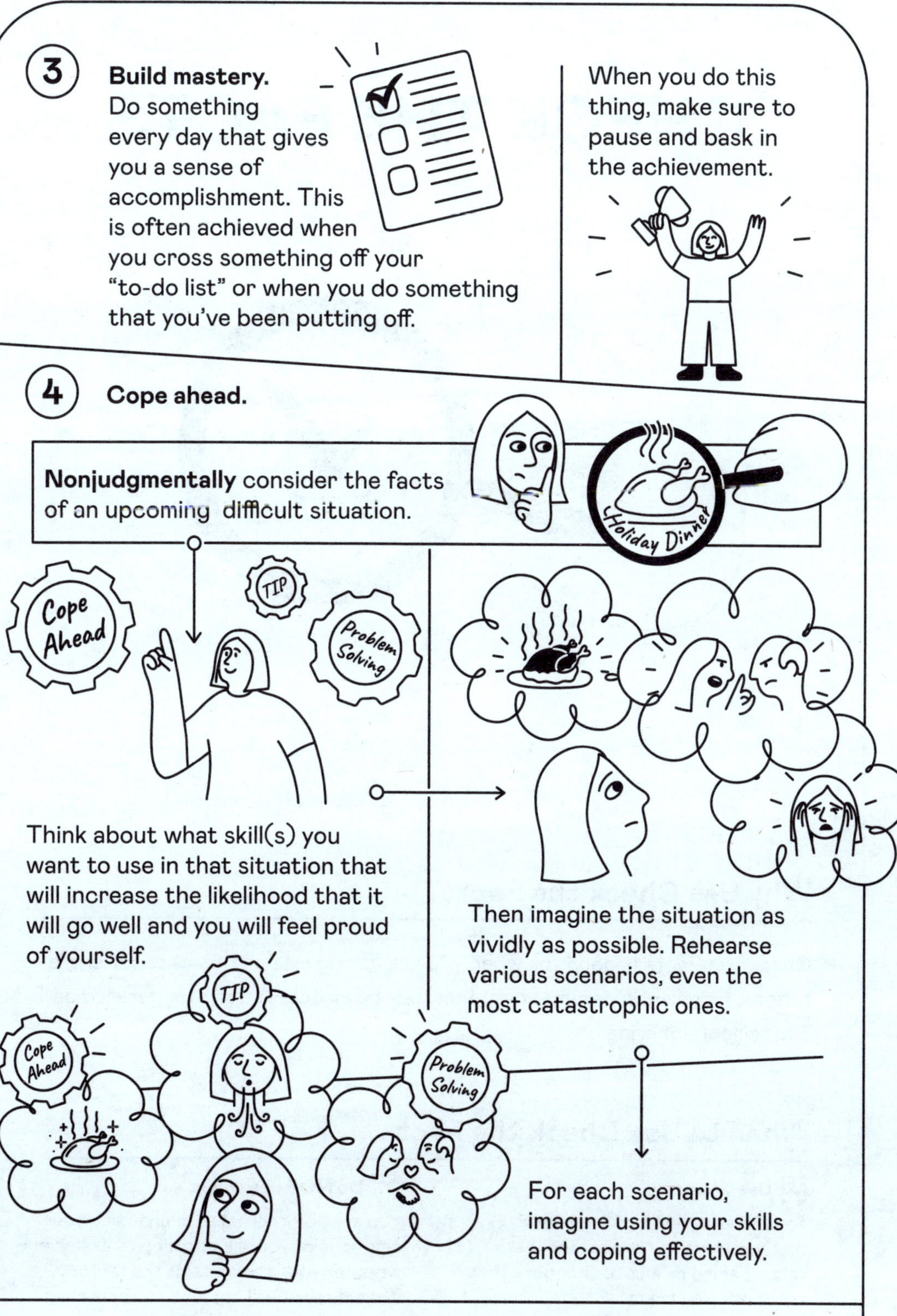

3 **Build mastery.** Do something every day that gives you a sense of accomplishment. This is often achieved when you cross something off your "to-do list" or when you do something that you've been putting off.

When you do this thing, make sure to pause and bask in the achievement.

4 **Cope ahead.**

Nonjudgmentally consider the facts of an upcoming difficult situation.

Think about what skill(s) you want to use in that situation that will increase the likelihood that it will go well and you will feel proud of yourself.

Then imagine the situation as vividly as possible. Rehearse various scenarios, even the most catastrophic ones.

For each scenario, imagine using your skills and coping effectively.

When ABC isn't effective, practice these skills:

WISE MIND · DISTRACT · IMPROVE

CHECK THE FACTS

Why Use Check the Facts?

Check the Facts is good for when you are having lots of thoughts (interpretations, judgments, assumptions) that may be inaccurate or exaggerated and add to your suffering.

When to Use Check the Facts

☑ **Use when:**

You are experiencing an emotion that you want to change, and it's accompanied by lots of thoughts that are causing distress.

☒ **Do NOT use when:**

You are not interested in changing your emotions or you are unwilling to examine whether your thoughts fit the facts. That mindset will not lead to accurate assessment of your thoughts.

CHECK THE FACTS is a skill designed to help you change an unwanted emotion by checking whether it fits the facts of the situation (or whether it's based on inaccuracies, assumptions, or judgments). Essentially, Check the Facts is a strategy from cognitive therapy that is used to help understand the connection between thoughts and feelings. Determining whether your emotional reaction fits the facts of the situation and, if it doesn't, working to change your thoughts and interpretations, can lead you to experience a change in how you're feeling.

The skill involves identifying your interpretations and emotion in response to a prompting event and then determining whether those thoughts and emotions make sense and thus "fit the facts" of the situation. It's separating factual thoughts from interpretations, assumptions, or "catastrophizing" (assuming the worst).

If your interpretations don't fit the facts of the situation, then it's likely that changing them will influence your emotion in a significant way. For example, if your initial thought about a friend not calling you back is "they must hate me for something I did," you are likely to feel shame and regret. If you check the facts, you might remember that this friend often doesn't call you back in a timely manner and that the last time you were together, you had a good time. So you might revise your interpretation to "I'm disappointed that she hasn't called me back yet." This new interpretation would be associated with some disappointment that feels more manageable.

If our thoughts and emotions do fit the facts, we can turn to problem solving or other skills to help with our emotional experience.

How to Know If Check the Facts Is Working

Check the Facts is working when you examine your thoughts and determine whether they fit the facts of the situation or not. Sometimes working through Check the Facts will lead to an "aha" moment where you realize that you've been thinking about a situation in an unhelpful way. This realization will open up new opportunities for skillful behavior.

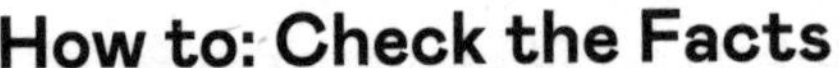

How to: Check the Facts

1 Use the **Model for Describing Emotions** to identify:

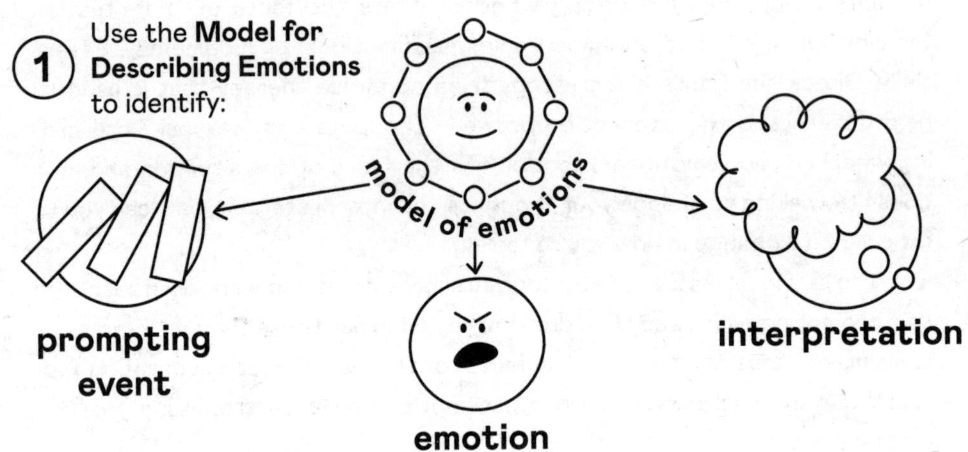

2 Write out, in detail, your **thoughts** and **interpretations** of the **prompting event**.

Interpretation One
Interpretation Two
Interpretation Three

Do you see any judgments? Do these interpretations assume a threat? Or a catastrophe?

For example

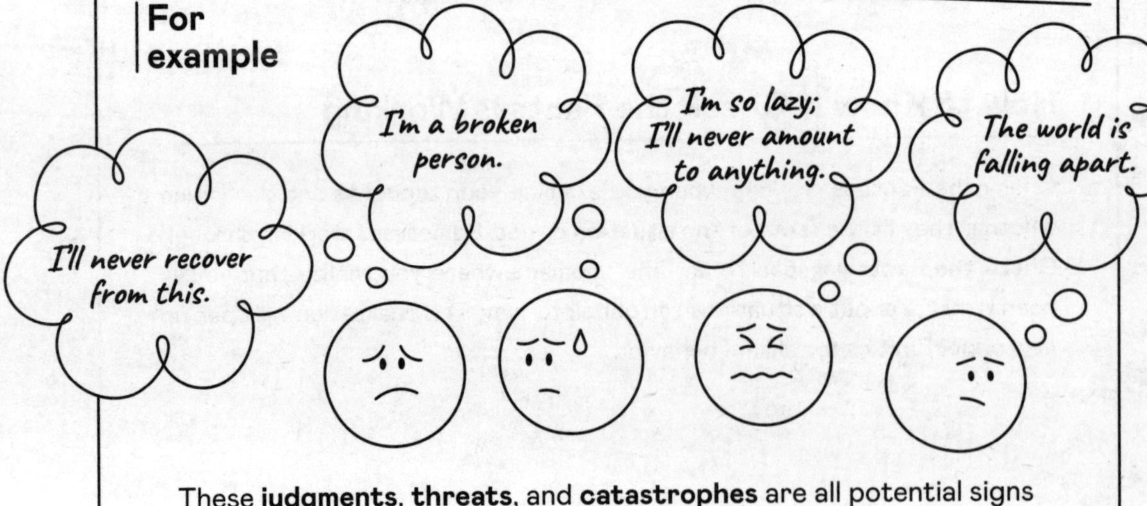

These **judgments**, **threats**, and **catastrophes** are all potential signs that your thoughts don't fit the facts of the situation.

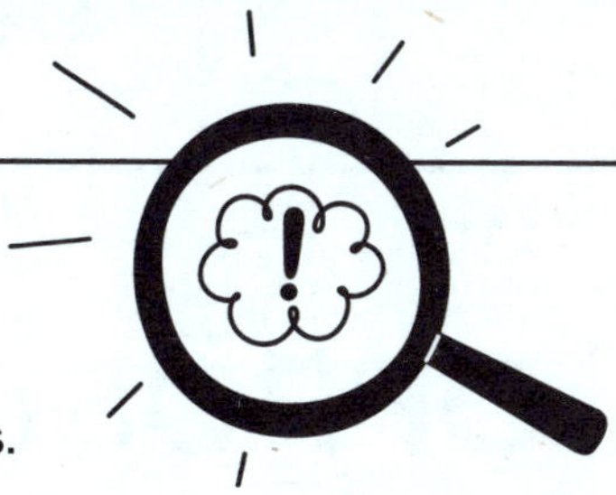

3 Use the mindfulness skill of **Describe** to rephrase your interpretations without judgments.

For example

I feel angry at myself right now.

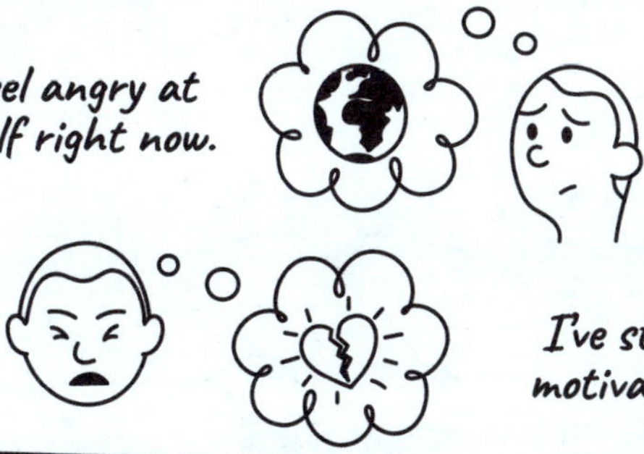

Things feel overwhelming in the world right now.

This feels really hard, and it may take time to recover.

I've struggled with motivation recently.

Using **Describe** to label your experience will often lessen the emotional pain.

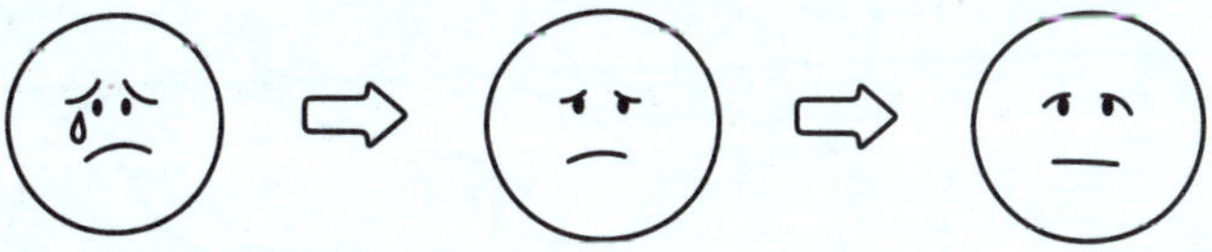

4 Look at your original interpretations and your revised interpretations.

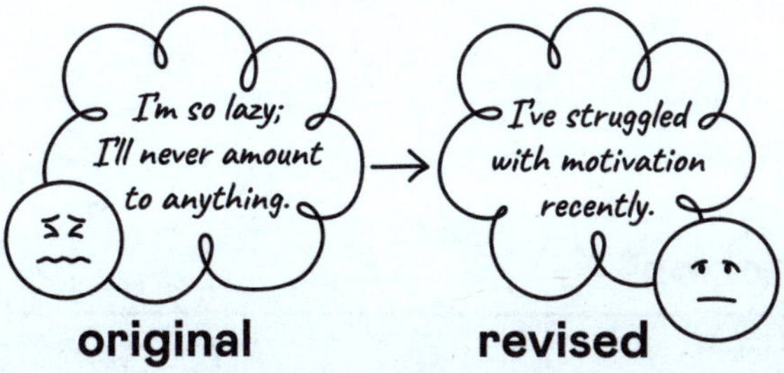

I'm so lazy; I'll never amount to anything. → *I've struggled with motivation recently.*

original **revised**

Ask yourself:

Which one fits the facts of the situation better?

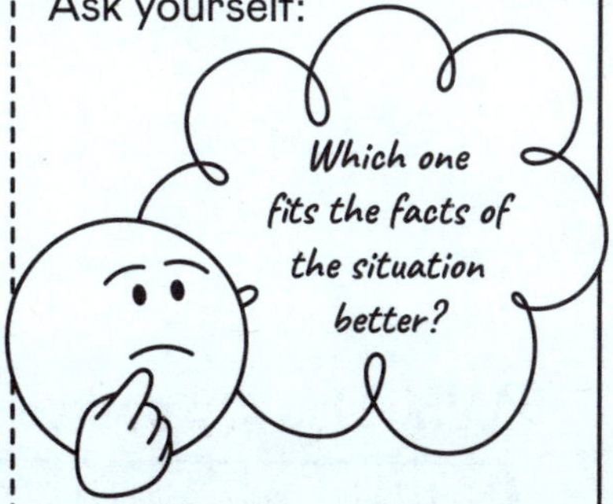

If it's your revised interpretation, update your Model and notice if a new emotion arises.

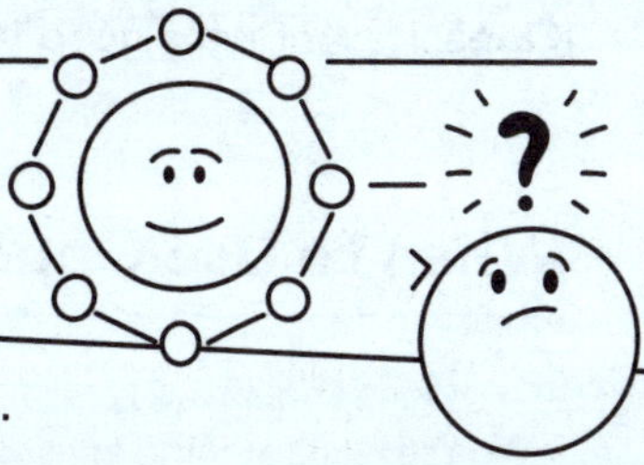

5 Even if your interpretations fit the facts...

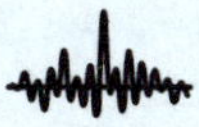

...the intensity of the emotion... **or** 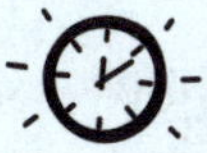 ...how long you're feeling the emotion...

may not fit the facts

...signaling it's time to try skills like **Opposite Action** or **Problem Solving.**

When Check the Facts isn't effective, practice these skills:

PROBLEM SOLVING · OPPOSITE ACTION

OPPOSITE ACTION

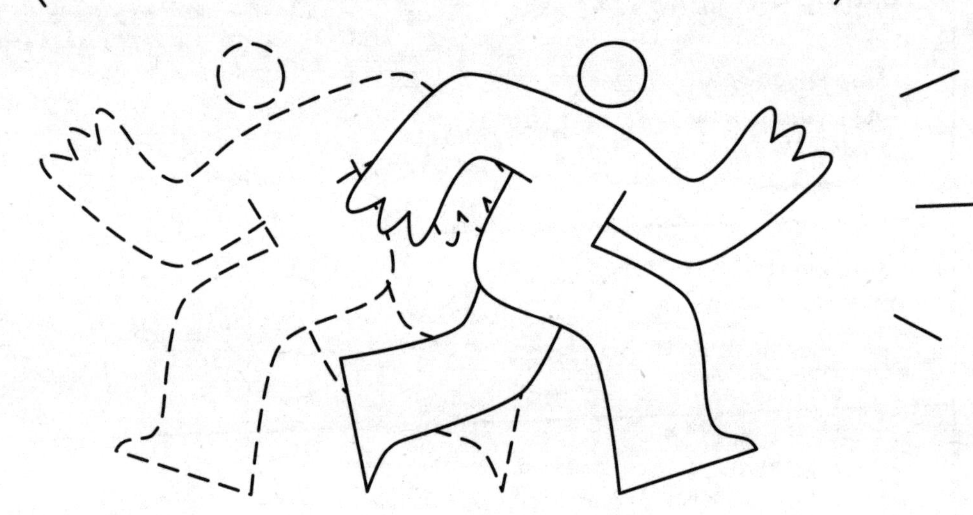

Why Use Opposite Action?

Opposite Action is good for when you want to change how you are feeling.

When to Use Opposite Action

☑ **Use when:**

- You're experiencing an emotion that you want to change.
- You're experiencing an emotion that's getting in the way of reaching one of your goals.
- You're having urges to avoid something that's important and/or needs doing.

☒ **Do NOT use when:**

The emotion is doing something important for you. For example, fear can help you avoid a legitimate danger. Or if you just experienced the death of a loved one, it's important to feel the sadness and grief rather than immediately try to change it.

OPPOSITE ACTION is all about changing how you feel by first changing your behavior. Typically, when we feel a certain way, we have urges to behave in ways that are consistent with that emotion—we call those "action urges." For example, when we feel fear, we often have urges to run away or avoid; when we feel sad, we often have urges to shut down and reduce energy output. Our action urges tend to be stronger the more intense the emotion. Opposite Action refers to counteracting what we are feeling by acting opposite to the urges we feel. It's similar to the concept "fake it 'til you make it."

For Opposite Action to work, it's important that you want to change how you're feeling and that you commit to doing it "all the way." If you are unwilling to change how you feel, it will be harder for you to engage in Opposite Action in an effective way. "All the way" refers to throwing yourself into the new behavior with mind, body, and soul. The key is to do the opposite action over and over until you notice that the intensity of the emotion has decreased, or the emotion has changed altogether. When we practice Opposite Action, we often get more active and engage in a new, more skillful behavior. In that way, Opposite Action can also lead to a sense of mastery or accomplishment.

Opposite Action works best when the emotion you want to change does not fit the facts or when the intensity or duration of the emotion is too high for the situation.

How to Know If Opposite Action Is Working

Opposite Action is working when the intensity of the original emotion starts going down. You may start to feel other emotions that are consistent with your opposite actions. Know that Opposite Action takes time—don't expect it to work within minutes. Instead, keep engaging in opposite actions all the way until your original emotion changes. If the intensity is not decreasing, then reconsider whether the emotion is doing something important for you.

How to: Opposite Action

1 Identify the emotion you're feeling and want to change (it's OK if it's imprecise or if you're having difficulty here).

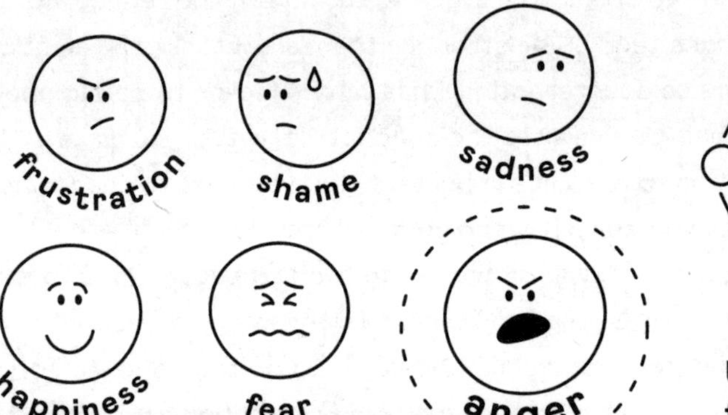

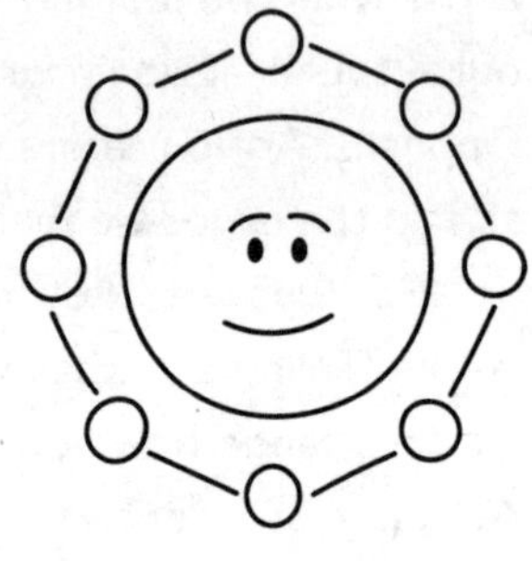

Use the **Model for Describing Emotions** to help.

2 Identify your action urges.

What does your emotion want you to do in this moment?

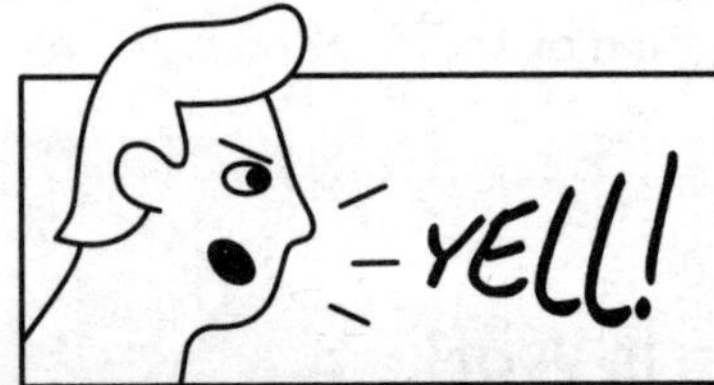

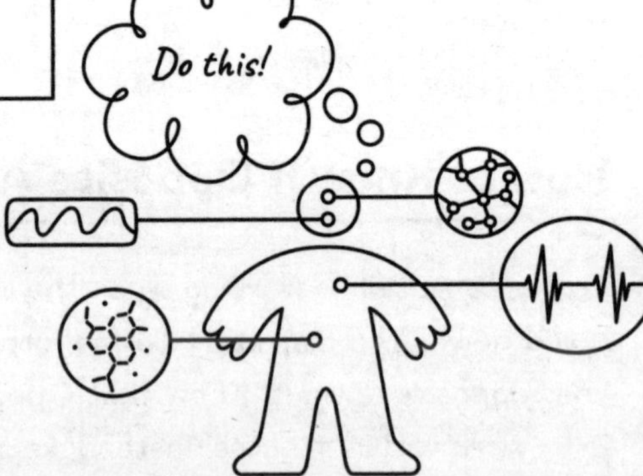

Urges can come in the form of physical sensations or thoughts.

3 Identify what the opposite of those urges would be in behaviors and thoughts.

avoid

approach

lash out

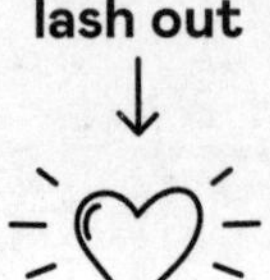

be kind

repeatedly reach out to someone

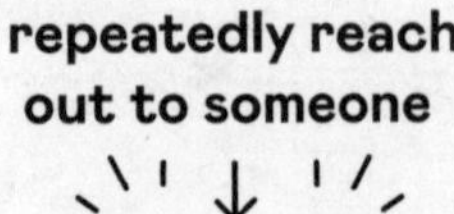

avoid

stay in bed

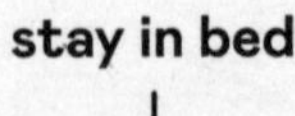

get active

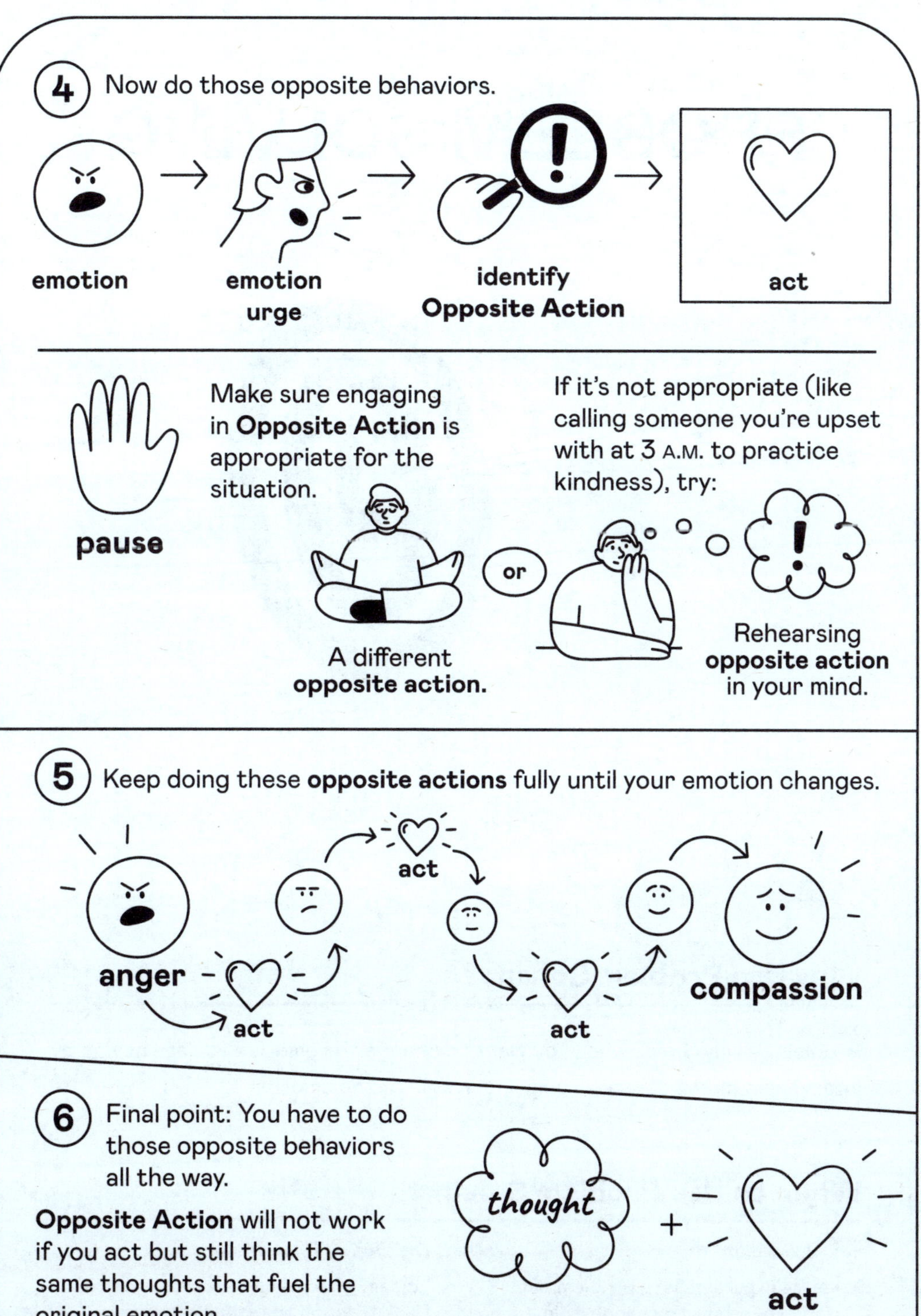

When Opposite Action isn't effective, practice these skills:

MINDFULNESS OF CURRENT EMOTIONS

RADICAL ACCEPTANCE · PROBLEM SOLVING

PROBLEM SOLVING

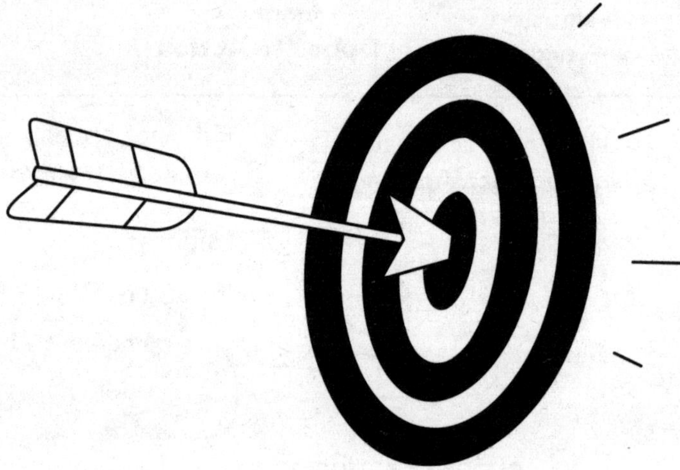

Why Use Problem Solving?

Problem Solving helps when you want to change the emotion you are having by intervening at the cause (prompting event) of the emotion.

When to Use Problem Solving

☑ **Use when:**

- You're experiencing a problem but don't know how to change it (in a skillful manner).
- You're having urges to address a problem in an impulsive way.

☒ **Do NOT use when:**

You are in crisis or too distressed to think through the steps in a clear-headed, Wise Mind manner. Use other skills first and then try Problem Solving.

PROBLEM SOLVING is a skill that breaks down the steps needed to effectively solve problems. If you can solve the problem that is eliciting emotions and difficulty for you, that is a great outcome. Some of us are natural problem solvers or have been taught how to problem solve by parents, caretakers, or teachers. Others of us were never taught or need to develop the skill. Don't despair if you feel like you don't know how to problem solve effectively—we are here to help!

The skill of Problem Solving involves going through a sequence of steps, outlined in the next pages, to arrive at potential solutions and then implementing one of those solutions. One benefit of practicing this skill is realizing there is always a solution to every problem. Realistically, it may not be an easy solution or one that will immediately work. But knowing that there is always a solution often opens up possibilities and moves us away from being stuck or overly pessimistic.

Problem Solving also teaches us how to be more flexible in our approach to problems and their solutions. Instead of getting stuck thinking there's only one way to approach something or that a problem is unsolvable, we learn how to brainstorm different options. A lot of these options will be other skills in this book. Incorporating mindfulness skills into the process also helps us see the problem more clearly, which leads to more appropriate solutions that are in line with our goals.

How to Know If Problem Solving Is Working

You put your plan into action and the problem is solved! Or, if the problem is a big one, you feel like you are steadily taking the right steps toward solving it.

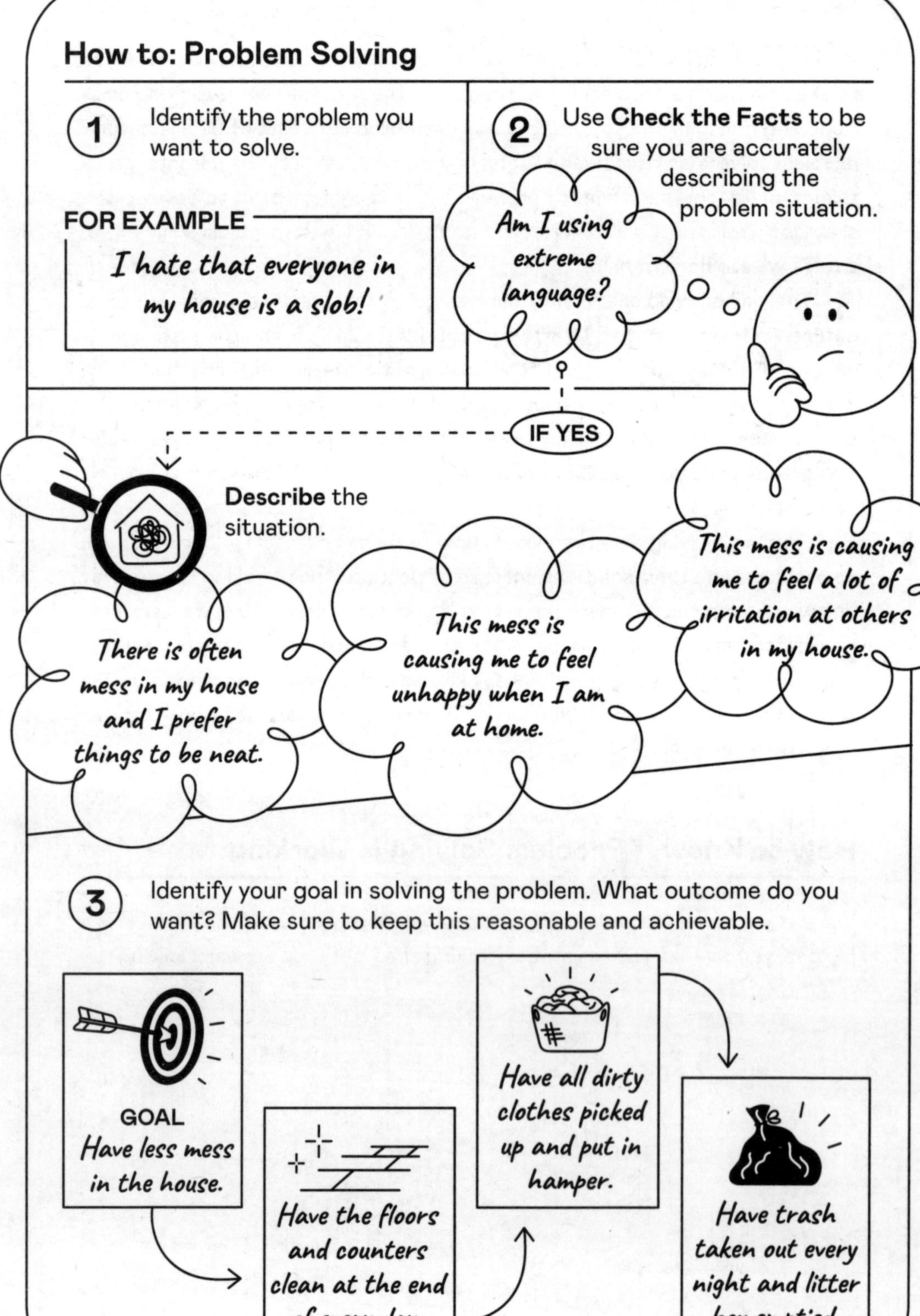
How to: Problem Solving
1 Identify the problem you want to solve.
FOR EXAMPLE
I hate that everyone in my house is a slob!
2 Use **Check the Facts** to be sure you are accurately describing the problem situation.
Am I using extreme language?
IF YES
Describe the situation.
There is often mess in my house and I prefer things to be neat.
This mess is causing me to feel unhappy when I am at home.
This mess is causing me to feel a lot of irritation at others in my house.
3 Identify your goal in solving the problem. What outcome do you want? Make sure to keep this reasonable and achievable.
GOAL
Have less mess in the house.
Have the floors and counters clean at the end of every day.
Have all dirty clothes picked up and put in hamper.
Have trash taken out every night and litter box emptied.

4

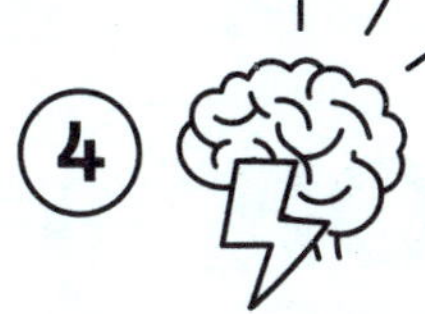

Brainstorm solutions. Come up with ALL the ways in which the goal might be reached. Don't censor at this point. The more, the better.

1 *Move out and live on my own.*

2 *Kill everyone and live on my own. (spoiler: this is NOT a recommended solution! We are including it n the spirit of demonstrating non-censorship!)*

3 *Ask them to clean up after themselves using DEAR MAN GIVE FAST.*

4 *Create a behavioral plan to reward cleanliness.*

5 *Do all the cleaning myself.*

6 *Do some (not all) cleaning myself to the point where it feels more tolerable.*

7 *Change how I think and feel about the mess so I'm no longer bothered by it.*

8 *Radically accept the mess.*

9 *Hire a daily housecleaner.*

5

Choose a solution that fits the goal and has a good chance of working. If unsure, do **Pros/Cons** of a couple different options to find the best one.

✗ *1, 2, 5, 7, 9 are not realistic or in line with my values.*

✗ *3 could work with my partner and teenage son, but not my toddler.*

✗ *4 could work but we already have other behavioral plans*

✓

That leaves 6 and 8. A combination of the two would be the best solution—clean the things that really bother me and radically accept the "smaller stuff."

6

Implement the solution by putting it into action.

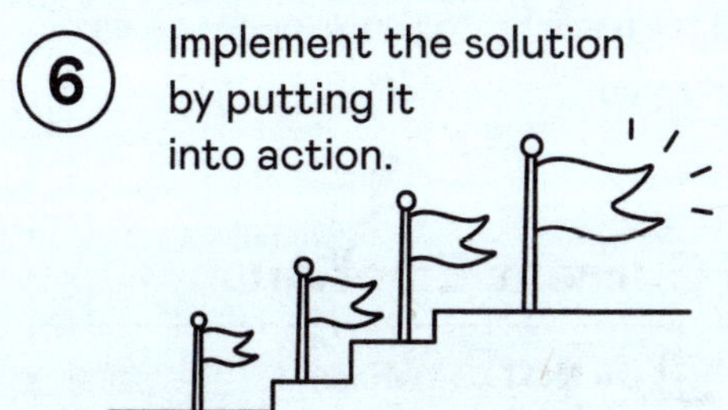

Break it down into steps and sequentially go through the steps.

7

Evaluate the results—did it work?

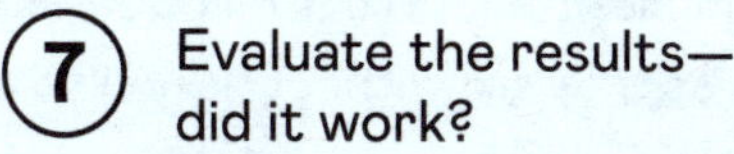

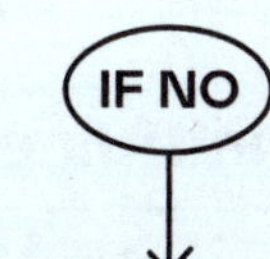

Go back to Step 5 and try a new solution.

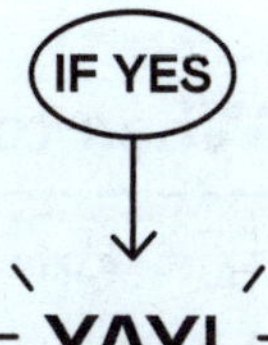

When Problem Solving isn't effective, practice these skills:

WISE MIND · RADICAL ACCEPTANCE · TIP

MINDFULNESS OF CURRENT EMOTIONS

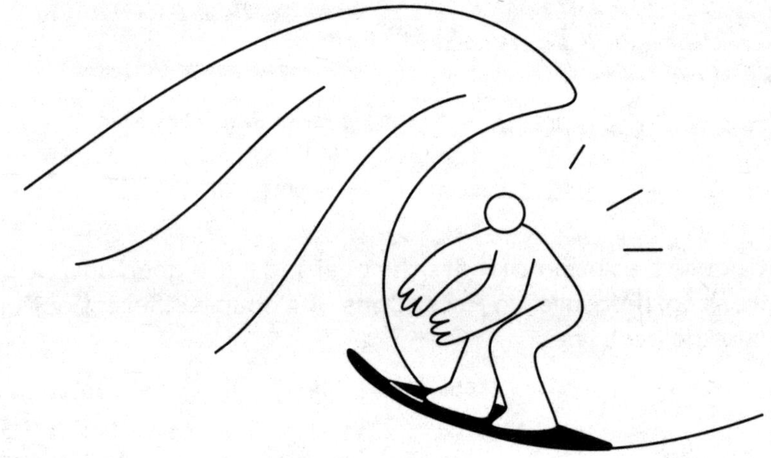

Why Use Mindfulness of Current Emotions?

Mindfulness of Current Emotions is good for learning to just experience emotions as they are without having to act on them.

When to Use Mindfulness of Current Emotions

☑ **Use when:**

- Almost always when emotions arise!
- Especially when you experience emotions that can't be avoided or changed in the moment.

☒ **Do NOT use when:**

You can't effectively control urges to engage in harmful or unwanted behaviors. When emotional intensity gets too high, you may want to consider other skills first.

MINDFULNESS OF CURRENT EMOTIONS is the skill of just experiencing your emotion without doing anything to try to avoid it, change it, or prolong it. It involves the mindfulness skills of Observe and Describe as well as Nonjudgmentally because you are noticing and labeling what you are experiencing without adding on or evaluating.

Often when we experience an intense, unpleasant emotion, we do ineffective things to get rid of it. We may try to avoid the emotion by mindlessly scrolling through our phone, or we may try to numb ourselves to the emotion with drugs or alcohol. We may reach out to someone and ask them to reassure us that we are a decent person. When we *only* focus on escaping difficult emotions, we don't have the opportunity to learn that the emotion will not destroy us and that it will eventually change on its own. This is actually quite miraculous to contemplate! No emotion lasts forever! Practicing Mindfulness of Current Emotions involves being a scientist with our own emotional experience.

Mindfulness of Current Emotions is also a generally important life skill. The truth is, no matter how much we effectively practice all the other skills in this book, we cannot fully prevent the experience of intense or uncomfortable emotions. Emotions are a part of life, and learning how to just experience them may paradoxically end up making them less intense and easier to tolerate. With practice, we can even learn to love our emotions and value them for what they communicate to us and how they keep us alive and in relationships.

How to Know If Mindfulness of Current Emotions Is Working

Like all mindfulness skills, it "works" when you practice it and notice what your emotion feels like. When you practice Mindfulness of Current Emotions, you will start to observe that your emotions will change without doing anything intentionally to change them.

How to: Mindfulness of Current Emotion

1 Start by asking yourself, what am I feeling in this moment? Name the emotion(s) that you notice.

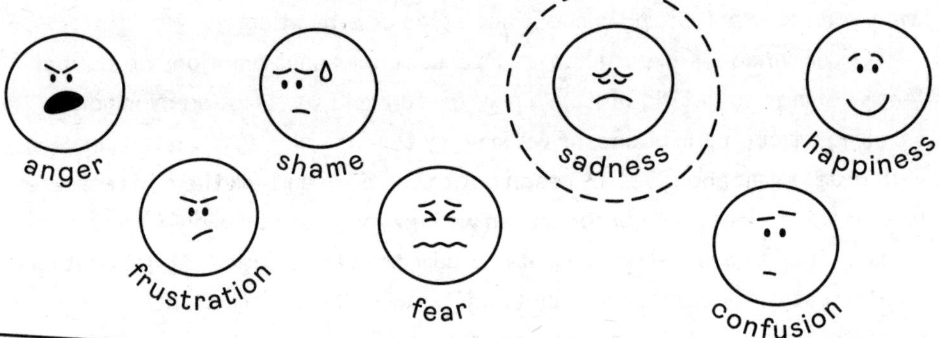

2 Observe your emotion by noticing how it shows up in your body.

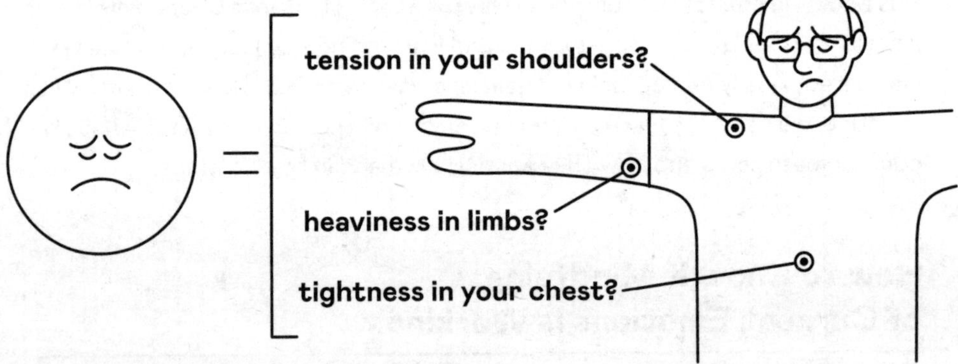

Without judgment, simply observe these sensations. See if you can watch them with curiosity rather than fear and resentment.

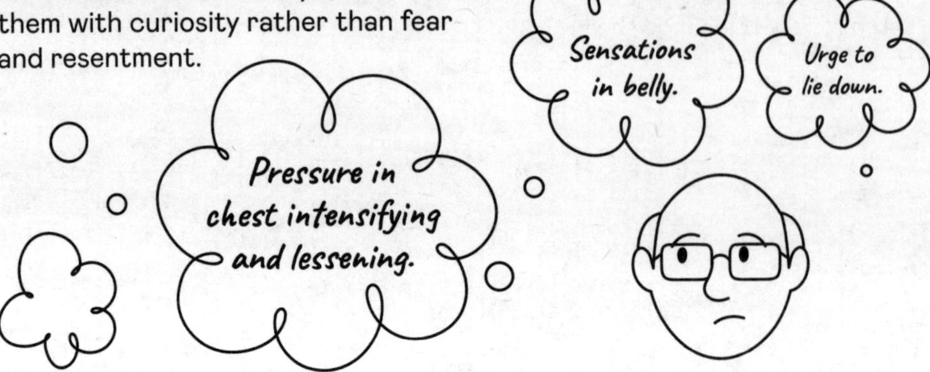

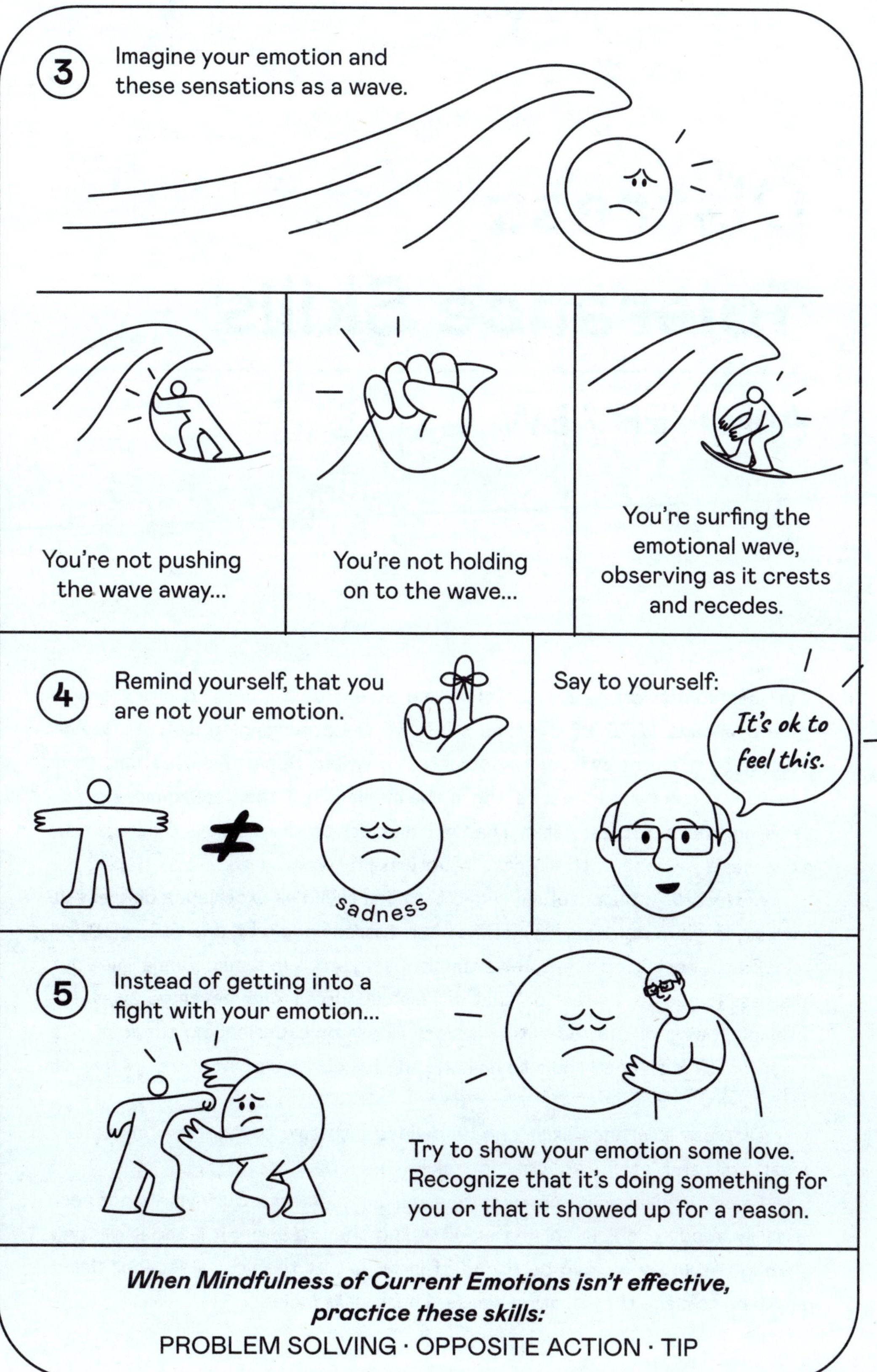
3
Imagine your emotion and these sensations as a wave.
You're not pushing the wave away...
You're not holding on to the wave...
You're surfing the emotional wave, observing as it crests and recedes.
4
Remind yourself, that you are not your emotion.
sadness
Say to yourself:
It's ok to feel this.
5
Instead of getting into a fight with your emotion...
Try to show your emotion some love. Recognize that it's doing something for you or that it showed up for a reason.
When Mindfulness of Current Emotions isn't effective, practice these skills:
PROBLEM SOLVING · OPPOSITE ACTION · TIP

Distress Tolerance Skills

AN OVERVIEW

Distress tolerance refers to tolerating stressful, distressing situations in effective ways. Much of the time, when we are experiencing distress, we do something to run away from it as quickly as possible. Some of these short-term "solutions" can help us feel better in the moment but then cause more problems, and more distress, later. The DBT distress tolerance skills teach us how to manage, or cope, with distress in more skillful ways.

Distress is a purposefully vague term here. We all experience distress at varying levels in our lives. Sometimes our distress could be due to a relatively minor and short-lived event, for example, being stuck in traffic. Sometimes our distress is due to a situation that will last a long time or never go away, for example, being diagnosed with a severe illness or experiencing the loss of a loved one. We all need tools to manage the full continuum of stressful events in our lives.

Distress tolerance skills can be divided into two categories: "crisis survival" skills and "reality acceptance" skills.

Crisis survival skills help us survive difficult moments. Surviving is not necessarily about problem solving or changing the situation; it's about getting through in a way we can be proud of later. Or, at the very least, not doing anything to make the situation worse. These skills include:

- The TIP skills for managing *extreme* distress, when we can't even think straight.
- The Distract skills for learning to temporarily distract from what's distressing us.
- The IMPROVE skill for helping make the current challenging moment better in some way.
- The Self-Soothe skill for learning how to be kind and soothing toward ourselves during difficult moments.
- The Pros/Cons skill to determine the best way to respond to a crisis.

Crisis survival skills aren't meant to solve long-term problems; instead, they are designed to help us more effectively navigate intense situations. They can be incredibly helpful when you need quick relief, but they have their limitations. If the only way we ever responded to difficult life events was to practice Crisis Survival skills, our problems would likely continue to build up over time. Using Crisis Survival skills in all difficult situations can also make us feel like we are constantly rushing to put out fire after fire, which is detrimental to our long-term health and wellness. We need other kinds of skills to help us manage difficult experiences in a more effective long-term manner. This is where reality acceptance skills come in.

Reality acceptance skills help us learn how to accept the reality of our lives so that we don't feel so distressed at every turn. They include:

- Radical Acceptance, which teaches us how to practice fully accepting the moment *exactly as it is.*
- Willingness, which teaches us how to practice being more willing to accept, rather than reject, reality.

All together, the DBT distress tolerance skills will help you get through life's difficult moments.

TIP

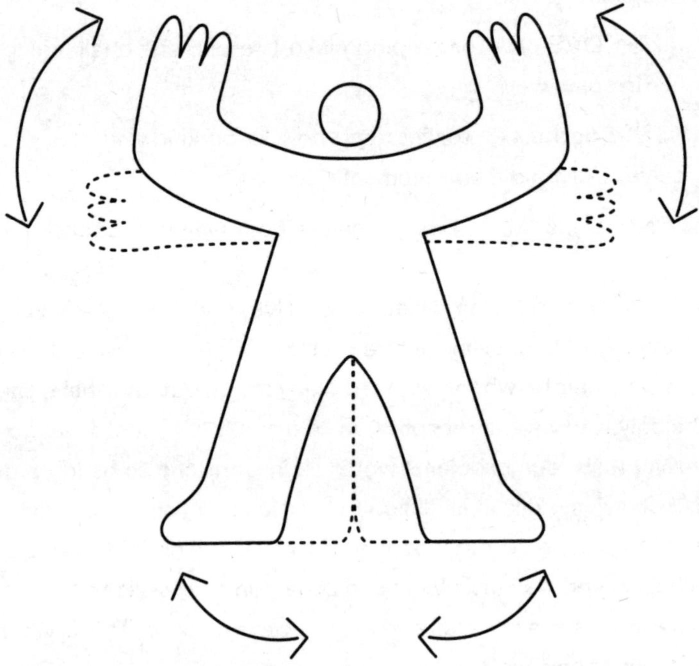

Why Use TIP?

TIP is helpful when your emotions are so intense or out of control that you can't think straight. The TIP skills are good for lowering your physiological arousal enough so that you can use other skills for the situation you're in.

When to Use TIP

☑ **Use when:**

You're in Emotion Mind, and your emotion or stress is so intense that you can't even think straight.

☒ **Do NOT use when:**

You're not in a state of high dysregulation or emotional intensity.

THE TIP skills are designed to reduce emotional distress quickly. They work by changing body chemistry so that we can proceed effectively or use other skills. There are four TIP skills:

- T Temperature: This skill activates the "mammalian dive reflex" by using cold water to trick your brain into thinking you're swimming under water. The dive reflex leads to automatic activation of the parasympathetic nervous system, lowering your heart rate and increasing blood flow to the brain and heart. If your brain thinks your body has been plunged into cold water, the dive reflex reactions will have a calming effect.
- I Intense exercise: When you feel extreme emotions or extreme stress, your body is actually quite revved up. Intense exercise can release some of the stress so that you feel calmer afterward. This is different from daily exercise; here, you are doing something that gets your heart rate up high and quickly. It could be doing something for just 30 seconds, or longer if you have the time.
- P Paced breathing: If you pace your breathing in a very particular way, you can slow down your heart rate and decrease emotional intensity. Often when we are upset, other people tell us to "just breathe." However, there are ways of breathing that are more likely to lead to less agitation and paced breathing is one such method.
- P Paired (or Progressive) muscle relaxation: This skill involves going through your body, muscle group by muscle group, first tensing the muscles as tight as you can and then releasing that tension. If you first tense your muscles really tightly before relaxing, you actually end up in a more relaxed state than if you just try to relax your muscles without tensing first.

Each of the TIP skills is designed to help lessen the intensity of your emotions.

How to Know If TIP Is Working

TIP skills are not designed to eliminate your emotions or solve the problem at hand. Instead, they are working when your extreme emotional intensity moves to only moderate intensity, so that you can use other skills.

How to: TIP Skills

 **Temperature:**

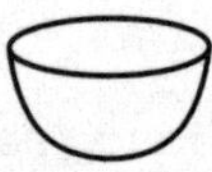

Get a large bowl that you can fit your entire face in.

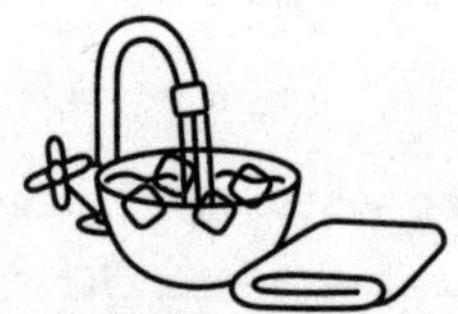

Fill the bowl with cold water and some ice. Have a towel nearby.

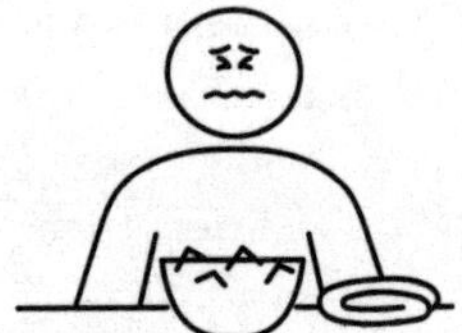

Place the bowl at waist level or lower so that when you bend over, its like diving downward.

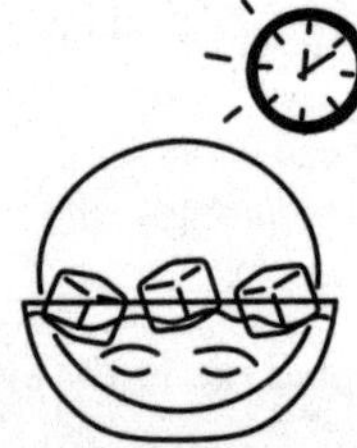

Hold your breath and plunge your face into the water. Hold for up to 30 seconds.

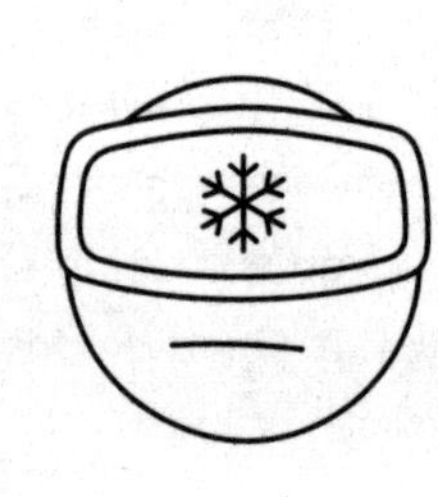

If you do not have access to a bowl of ice water, you can use an ice pack. Place the ice pack across your eyes and temple area and lower your head to below your heart. Hold your breath for up to 30 seconds.

 If you have a heart condition or take beta-blockers, consult a doctor first before you use the **Temperature** skill.

 **Intense exercise:** Do any intense physical exercise for as long as you can. Even 30 seconds can make a difference.

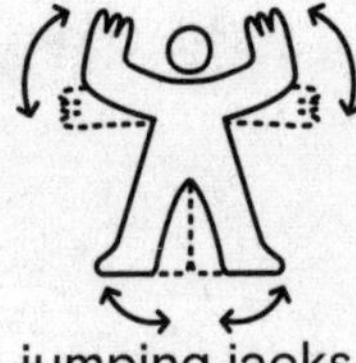

jumping jacks

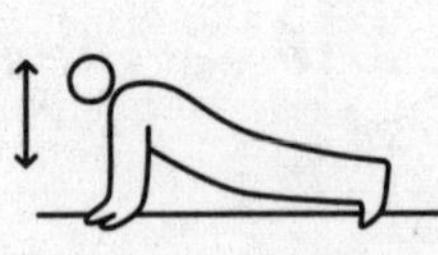

push-ups

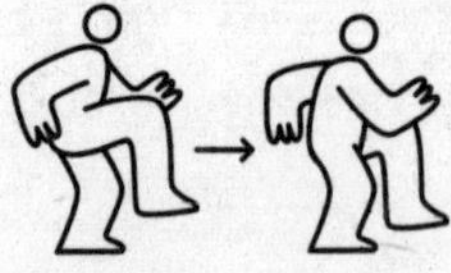

high-knees

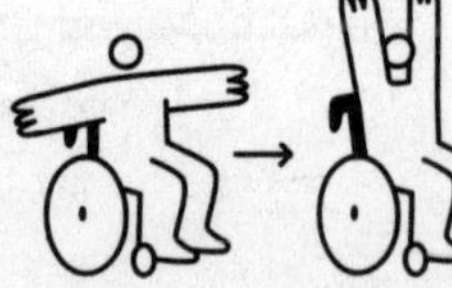

seated exercises

The goal is to get your heart rate up fast so that when you're finished, you come down to a more relaxed state.

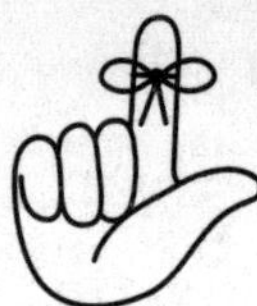

Remember: This skill isn't about getting in shape—it's about using short bursts of intense physical activity to help change your body chemistry.

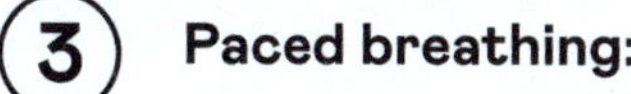

3 Paced breathing:

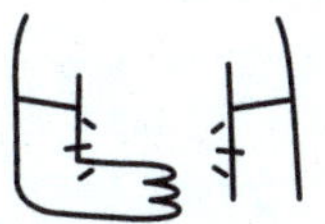

Breathe from your belly, not your chest.

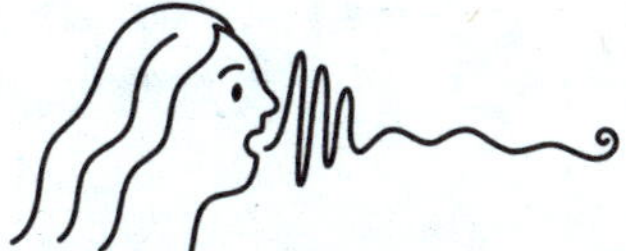

Slow down your rate of breathing.

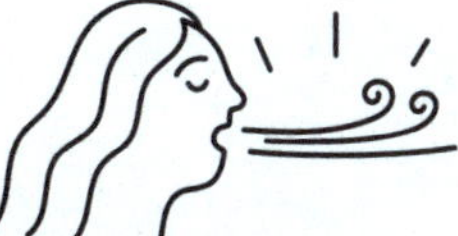

Make the exhale longer than your inhale.

Try:

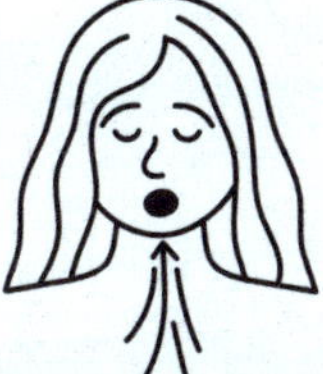

inhale for a count of 4 seconds

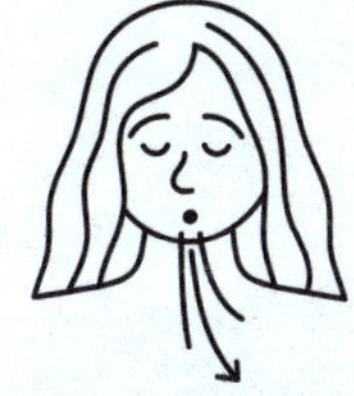

exhale for a count of 6 seconds

If your natural slow breathing rhythm is longer or shorter than 10 seconds, adjust accordingly.

4 Paired muscle relaxation:

While breathing in, deeply tense your body muscles as tight as you can.

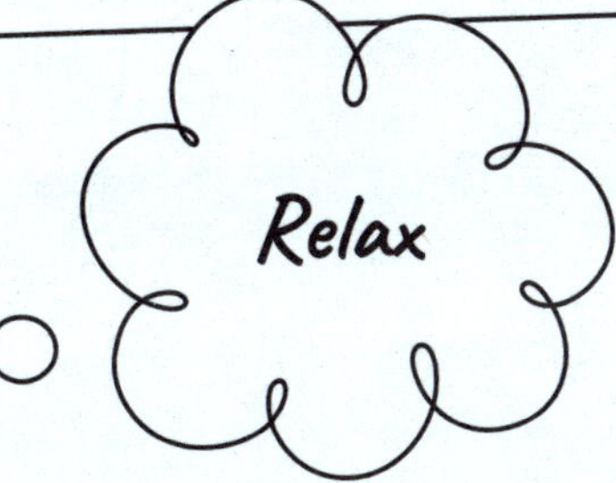

While breathing out, let go of the tension saying the word **relax** in your mind.

You can do this with your entire body...

...or you can go muscle group by muscle group.

face

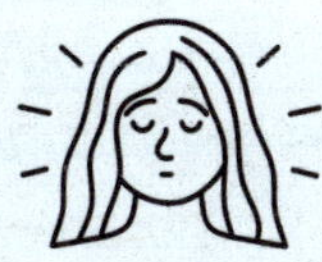

clench ⟶ relax

fist

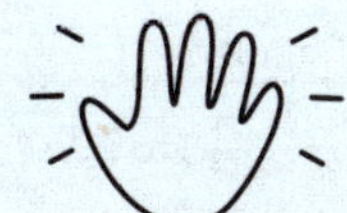

clench ⟶ relax

shoulders

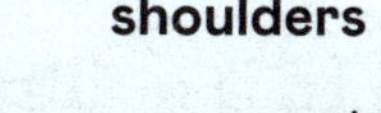

clench ⟶ relax

When TIP isn't effective, practice these skills:

PROBLEM SOLVING · MINDFULNESS OF CURRENT EMOTIONS

DISTRACT

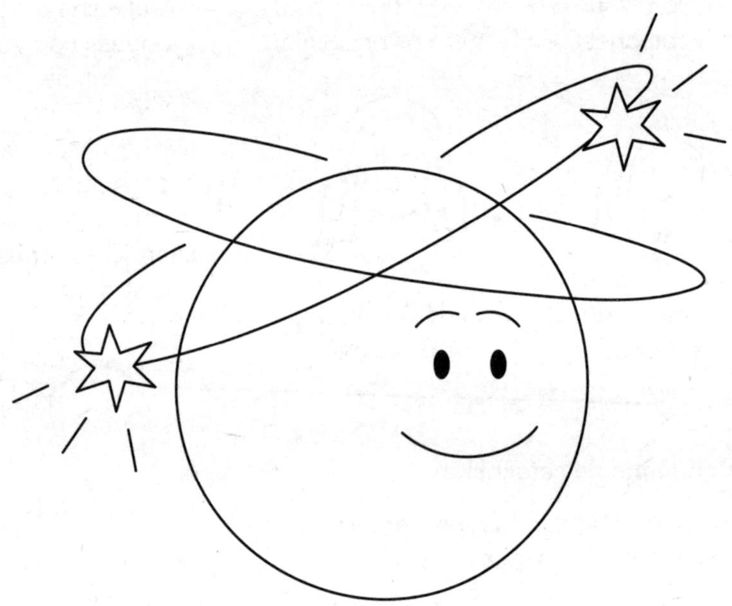

Why Use Distract?

Distract helps you get through a difficult situation without making it worse and helps you tolerate painful events and emotions when you cannot make them better right away.

When to Use Distract

☑ Use when:

You're experiencing a difficult situation that you can't solve or fix right away AND when it will not be damaging for you to take a bit of a "time out."

☒ Do NOT use when:

- The problem can be solved and avoidance is actually making the problem worse.
- You find that you use Distract for too long or that you always use it as your "go to" skill. Distract is to be used in short-term ways.

DISTRACT is a form of short-term skillful avoidance; you mindfully and effectively choose to step away from the crisis. This is different from burying your head in the sand and pretending the crisis doesn't exist. Distract is a skill set of seven strategies that you can remember with the acronym ACCEPTS.

- A Activities: Putting your full attention on something completely different (using the skill of Participate) to get your mind off the distressing situation.
- C Contributing: Doing something nice for someone else to take the focus off your problems. It could be something small, like telling someone you appreciate them, or much larger, like volunteering at a local charity.
- C Comparison: Comparing your situation to other worse situations, or comparing now to a time when you weren't coping as well.
- E Emotions: Doing something that elicits a different emotion than what you're currently feeling. Importantly, this doesn't need to mean replacing a negative emotion with a positive one. Just any different emotion than what you're feeling.
- P Pushing away: Getting what's distressing you out of your mind. This is mentally putting what's difficult in a metaphorical box, on a shelf, deep in a closet. Do this for a length of time that allows you to focus on something else, but don't forget to return to it later to problem solve!
- T Thoughts: Directing your mind to another mental activity that is incompatible with all the stressful, anxious thoughts you're having.
- S Sensations: Engaging in activities that elicit other strong sensations that don't cause harm to yourself.

How to Know If Distract Is Working

Distract is effective when you get through the crisis without doing anything to make it worse or without engaging in problematic behaviors.

How to: Distract

DISTRACT is a set of strategies for when you need to get your mind off something.

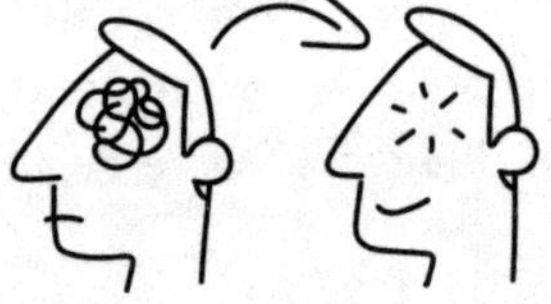

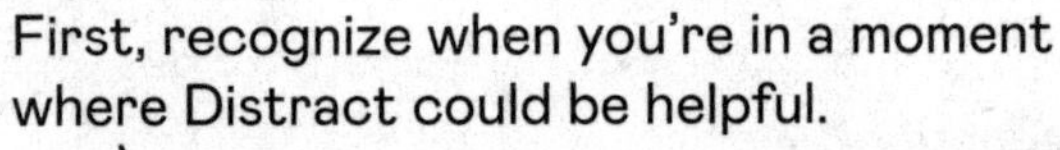

First, recognize when you're in a moment where Distract could be helpful.

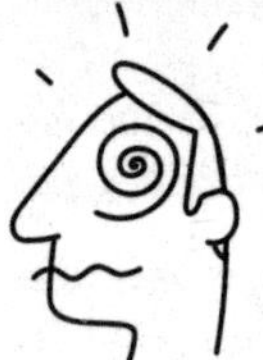

Like when you're ruminating...

...or when you have strong urges to engage in a problematic behavior.

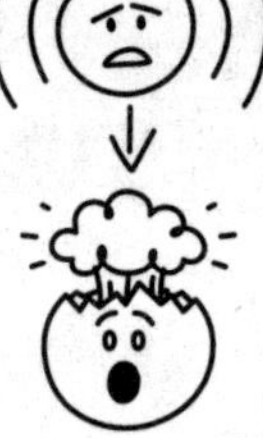

(A) ACTIVITIES

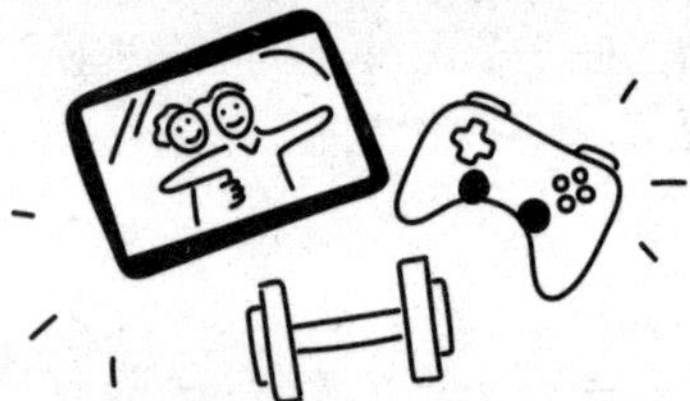

Put your attention on a completely different **Activity**.

Watch a video or movie, play a board game or video game, or engage in a sport or exercise. It could even be cleaning your room with your full attention.

(C) CONTRIBUTING

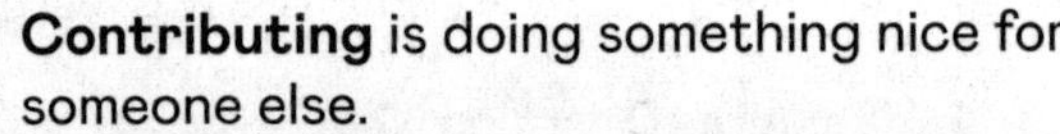

Contributing is doing something nice for someone else.

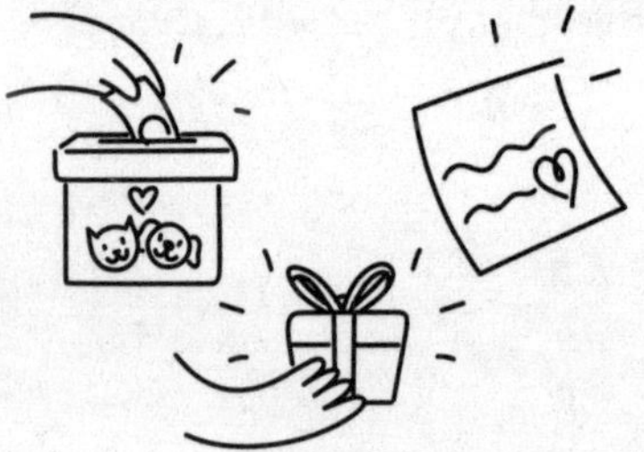

Volunteer, donate time or money to a favorite cause. Tell a close friend or family member something that you appreciate about them. Write a note or card to someone. Buy a small gift for somebody.

(C) COMPARISON

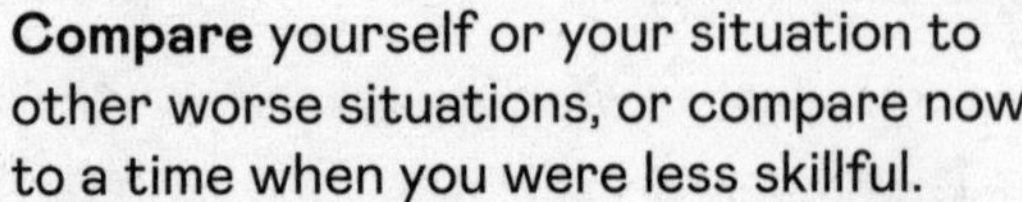

Compare yourself or your situation to other worse situations, or compare now to a time when you were less skillful.

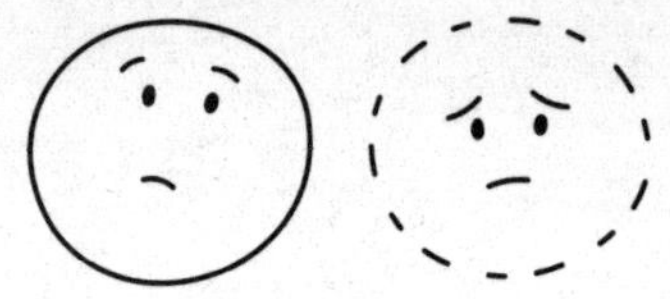

You can say to yourself, "This is hard AND I've gotten through worse," or "This is hard AND at least I have food and shelter, unlike others."

Ⓔ EMOTIONS

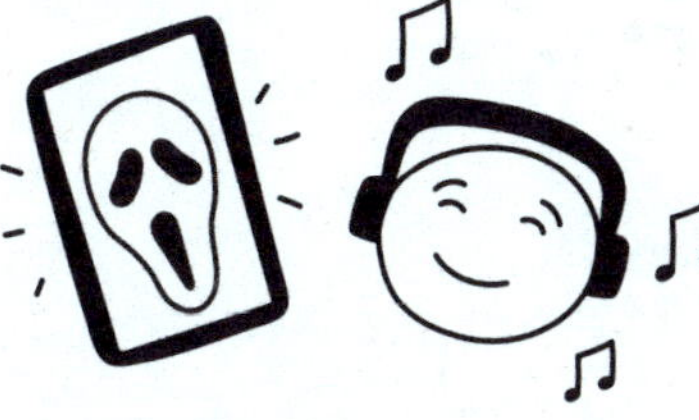

Emotions involve doing something that elicits a different emotion than what you're currently feeling.

Watch a very scary movie or a funny video, or listen to music that activates you in a different way.

Ⓟ PUSHING AWAY

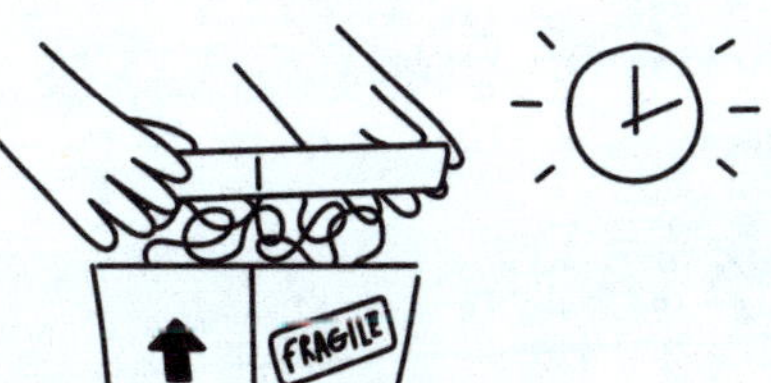

Pushing away is mentally putting what's difficult in a box, on a shelf, deep in a closet.

Say to yourself: "I'm not going to think about this at all for the next 15 minutes." Or "I'll return to this later, but for now, I have to focus on something else."

Ⓣ THOUGHTS

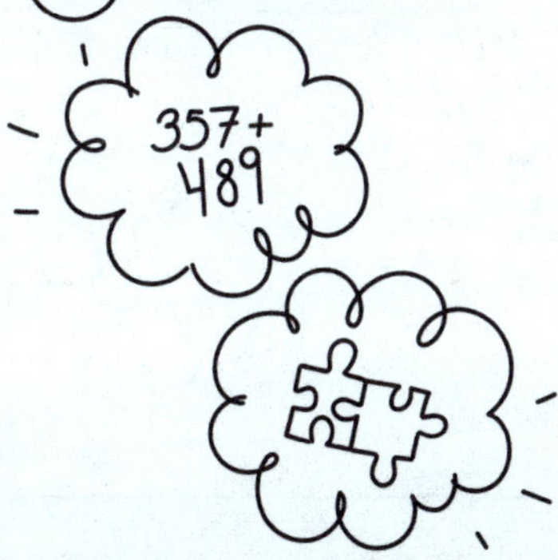

Direct your attention toward something that shifts your **thoughts** away from what's causing you distress. **Thoughts** include any mental activity that is incompatible with all your distressing thoughts.

Do subtraction or addition in your head. Try to remember all the lyrics of a song you like. Count the tiles in the ceiling in the room you're in. Count the number of trees that you see outside. Solve a puzzle.

Ⓢ SENSATIONS

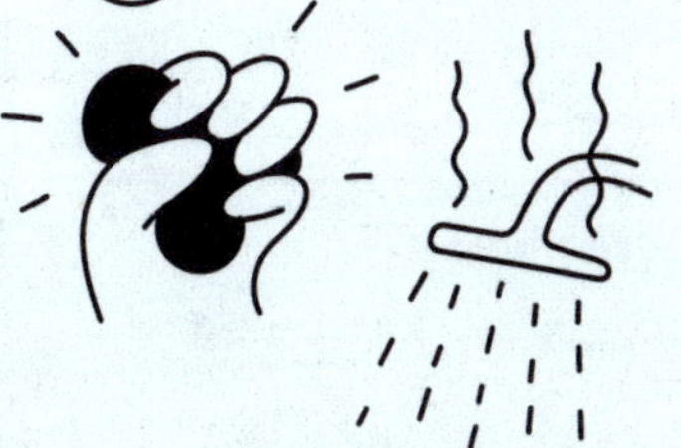

Engage in activities that elicit strong **sensations** to divert your mind from what is currently distressing you.

Hold ice, bite into a lemon, squeeze a stressball very hard, or take a very hot or very cold shower.

 Don't engage in sensations that cause you physical harm or pain.

When Distract isn't effective, practice these skills:

TIP · PROBLEM SOLVING

IMPROVE

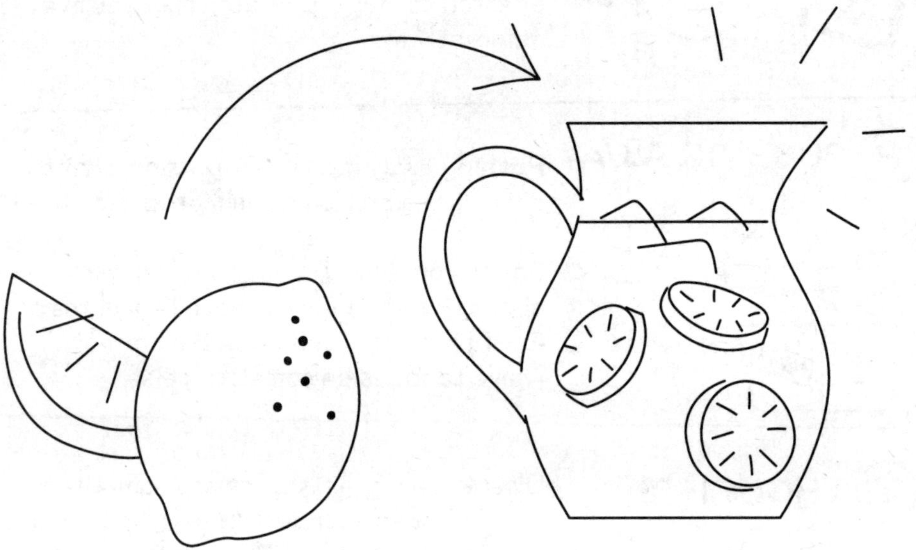

Why Use IMPROVE?

These skills are designed to make difficult moments better in some (usually small) way.

When to Use IMPROVE

☑ **Use when:**

You're experiencing a crisis or difficult moment that you can't solve or fix right away.

☒ **Do NOT use when:**

- The problem is solvable, and avoiding it makes the situation worse.
- You find that you use IMPROVE as your default approach to a crisis (which could get in the way of problem solving).

IMPROVE skills are about doing something with a crisis to lessen its severity in the moment. Similar to Distract, these skills are less about solving the immediate problem and more about coping more effectively. IMPROVE is an acronym that stands for seven strategies.

- I Imagery: Using visual imagery to create a more relaxing scene, your own personal image of a "happy place" that you bring to mind when you're feeling stressed.
- M Meaning: Making lemonade out of lemons—finding what meaning you can in this experience, even if it feels terrible. Often people find meaning through religious beliefs (for example, "God is testing me for a reason") but meaning can also be secular, like "I'll be a stronger person when I get through this."
- P Prayer: Asking for strength from a supreme being or greater wisdom to get through this difficult time. You may already incorporate prayer in your life. If not, you can pray to many things, including your Wise Mind.
- R Relaxation: Relaxing in some way to make this moment less painful. Think about something relaxing you can do for 5 minutes.
- O One thing in the moment: Putting your full attention into just one thing (anything!) that you're doing right in this moment. When we are experiencing high degrees of stress, our minds are usually in a thousand places at once.
- V Vacation: Giving yourself a brief mental and physical break. It's like getting into bed and pulling the covers up over your head for 20 minutes. You're saying to yourself: "I'm going to let myself zone out; when the timer goes off, my vacation is done, and I'm going back to work."
- E Encouragement: Essentially cheerleading yourself. This is repeating over and over things that you would probably say to someone else, but instead saying them to yourself: "You can do it!"

How to Know If IMPROVE Is Working

IMPROVE is effective when you get through the crisis and you feel like you've made the moment slightly more tolerable without engaging in problematic behaviors.

How to: Improve

IMPROVE is a collection of strategies to use when we want to lessen the severity of a crisis and/or make it better in some small way.

(I) IMAGERY

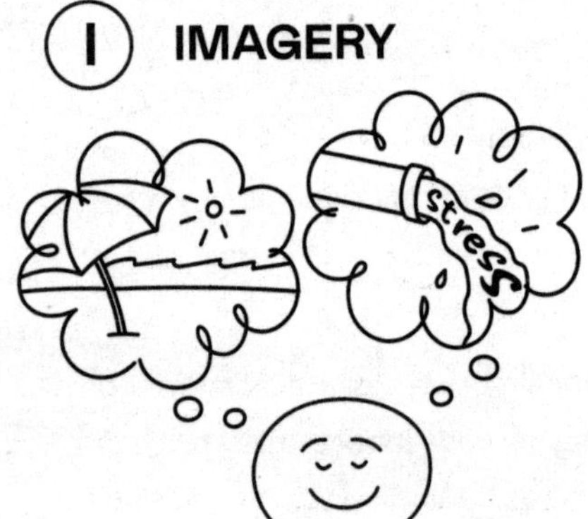

Use visual **imagery** to conjure a calm or relaxing scene.

Imagine your "happy place" or a tranquil natural paradise; imagine stress draining out of your body like water out of a pipe; imagine yourself as a superhero coping with this stress.

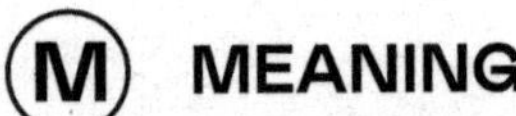

(M) MEANING

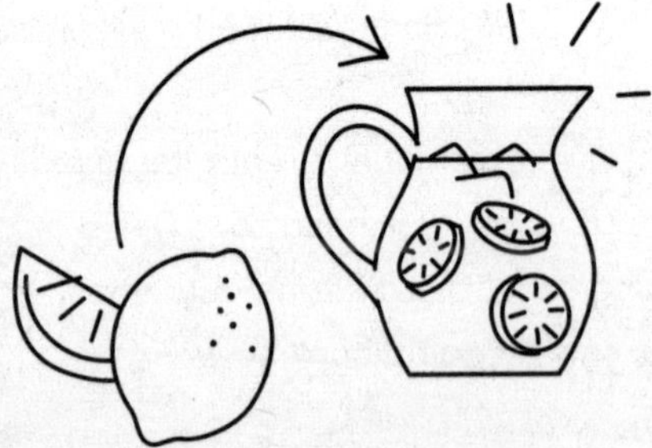

Think about what **meaning** you can take out of this experience. Make lemonade out of lemons.

"What doesn't kill me makes me stronger," "I'm learning something valuable here," "The reason I'm so upset is because this is important to me and that's good."

(P) PRAYER

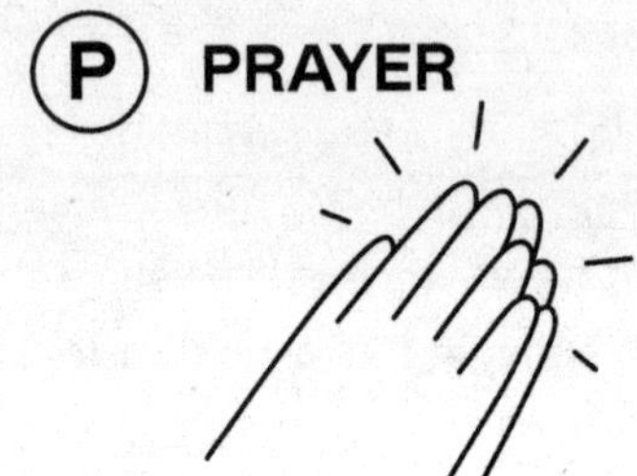

Open your heart to a greater wisdom and **pray** for strength and inner peace.

Pray to God or another supreme being or to your own **Wise Mind**. Ask for guidance, support, and love.

Ⓡ RELAXATION

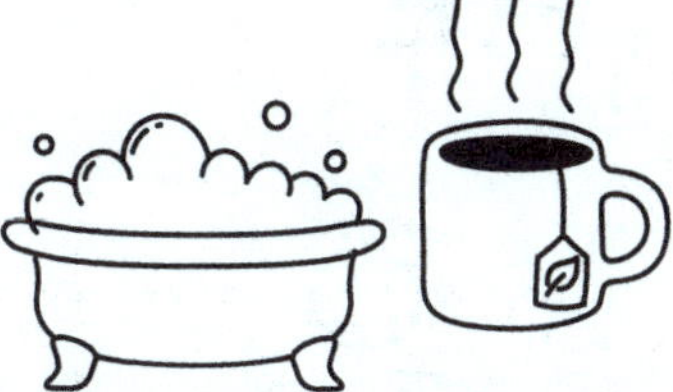

Relaxation helps calm your body and mind, reducing the stress of this current moment.

Take a calming bath or shower, sit and drink tea with a book in a comfy chair, do yoga stretching, or take a 5-minute time out to do something relaxing.

Ⓞ ONE THING IN THE MOMENT

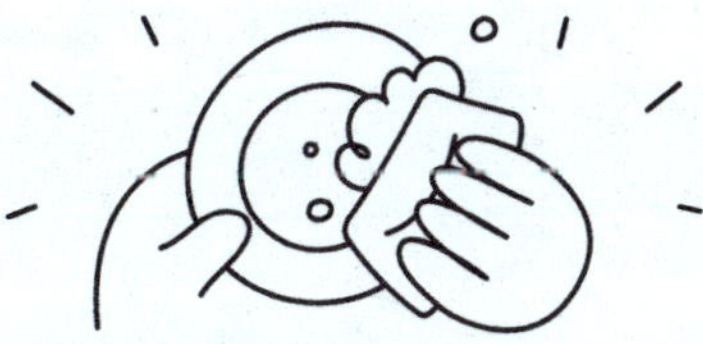

Immerse yourself fully in an activity, focusing all your attention on just that **one thing**.

If you're playing video games, focus entirely on the game. If you're washing dishes, concentrate solely on the act of washing—the feel of the water, the sound of the scrubbing, and the motion of your hands.

Ⓥ VACATION

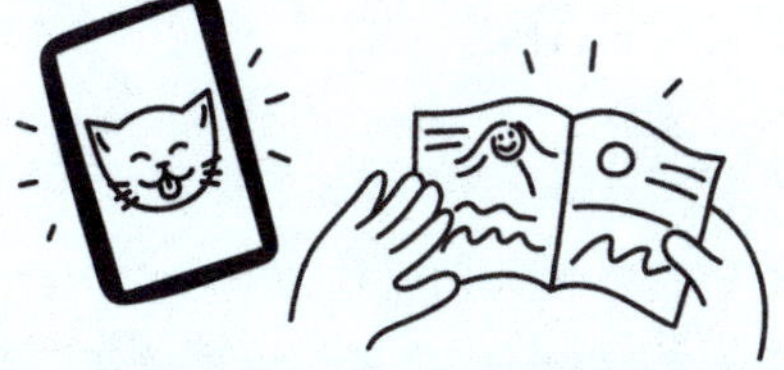

Give yourself a mental and physical break by taking a "**vacation**."

Look at the silliest stuff you can find online. Sit on the couch and eat chips for 15 minutes. Get into bed with a trashy novel or magazine for 20 minutes.

Ⓔ ENCOURAGEMENT

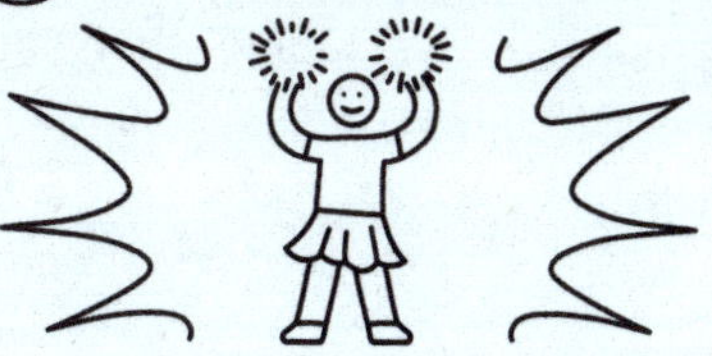

I can stand this. I can do this. I can cope with this. This won't last forever. This too shall pass. It's okay to feel this.

Be your own cheerleader. Use **Encouragement** to tell yourself that you have the strength to get through this hard time.

Write **IMPROVE** ideas when you're not in a crisis. That way, you don't have to use limited brain power when you're in a difficult moment to try to think of something helpful.

When IMPROVE isn't effective, practice these skills:

TIP · PROBLEM SOLVING

SELF-SOOTHE

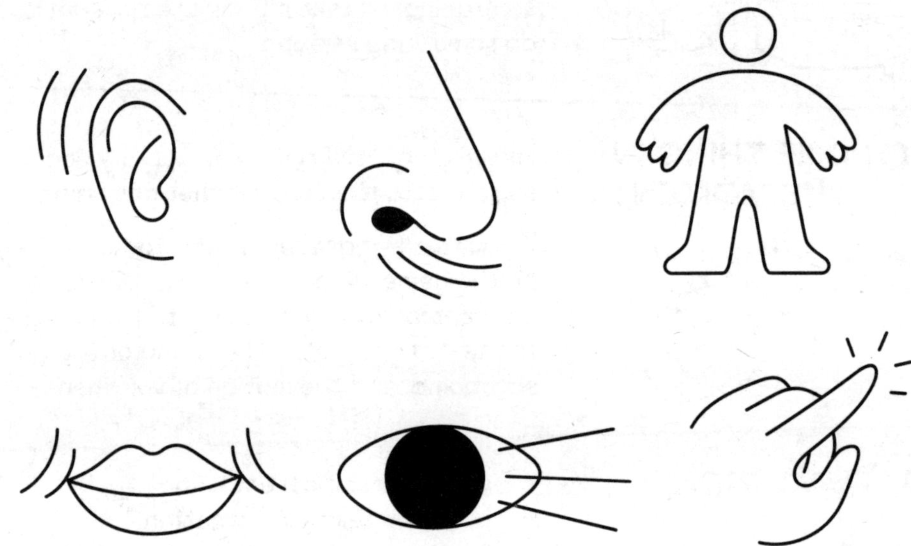

Why Use Self-Soothe?

The Self-Soothe skill is about being kind to yourself during times of stress. It's good for when you are in crisis or experiencing a difficulty, including when you are just having a bad day.

When to Use Self-Soothe

☑ **Use when:**

- You're experiencing difficulty that can't be solved right away.
- You are having urges to punish yourself for something you did or didn't do.
- You have had a bad day.

☒ **Do NOT use when:**

- You are using it to avoid doing something else that's hard.
- You find that you use Self-Soothe too much (that is, in place of other skillful behavior).

SELF-SOOTHE is a crisis survival distress tolerance skill. It refers to doing kind things for yourself, specifically by soothing the senses. It involves identifying items and activities that soothe you in each of your sense domains: sight, sound, taste, smell, and touch. During times of difficulty or crisis, you can engage with these items or activities as a way of soothing yourself, rather than criticizing or punishing yourself. It's treating yourself with the same degree of kindness that you would a loved one.

You can think of the five basic senses, plus the sense of the body, and generate a list of activities or items that bring you pleasure and promote an intent of being kind to yourself. For example, soothing yourself with taste could involve eating some of your favorite foods, drinking teas or other beverages that have strong and soothing flavors, or eating something from your childhood that you find comforting (in moderation). To soothe through hearing, you can put on calming music or music that you really love, or make a playlist of songs that all soothe you in a particular way. You can also listen to the sounds of nature. With smell, you can light a scented candle or attend to foods or cleaning products that have a nice scent. Or take a walk, and notice the smells of nature or fresh air. When it comes to your sense of sight, you can think about images that are soothing to you. You can look out a window, look at the night sky, find a picture of a painting online, look at photographs, or go for a walk and really take in your surroundings. Soothing through touch could include taking a long hot bath or shower, petting an animal, or putting lotion on and noticing how it feels on your skin. Finally, soothing the sense of your body could consist of some gentle movement like walking, yoga, or dancing.

As these examples indicate, Self-Soothe can be a very portable skill! Think of options that don't cost a lot of money or time to make them more likely to happen.

How to Know If Self-Soothe Is Working

As a crisis survival skill, Self-Soothe is "working" when you are tolerating the crisis without doing anything to make it worse. Since you are practicing being kind to yourself, you may also notice feelings of shame and/or guilt lessen or feelings of pleasure or enjoyment arise.

How to: Self-Soothe

1 Choose a sense (taste, hearing, smell, sight, touch, body) with which you want to practice.

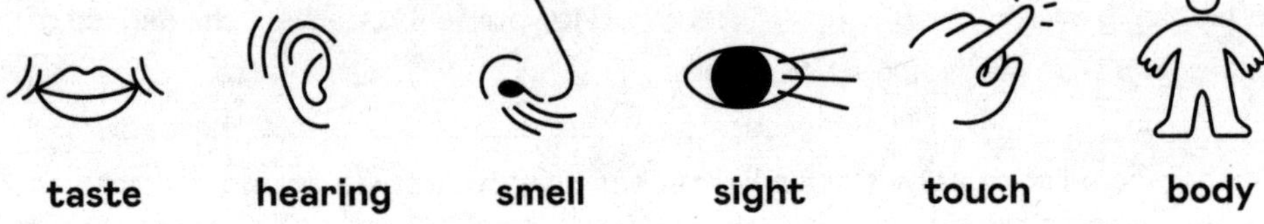

2 For each sense, identify something or many things that will soothe you. Consider trying something new.

taste	herbal tea	chocolate	fresh fruit
hearing	favorite songs	rain sounds	singing bowl
smell	favorite perfume	flowers	scented candle
sight	favorite tv show	photo of loved ones	nature
touch	fidget	knitting	hot bath
body	dancing	yoga	going for a walk

3. If self-soothing feels hard because you believe you don't deserve it, distract yourself from those thoughts.

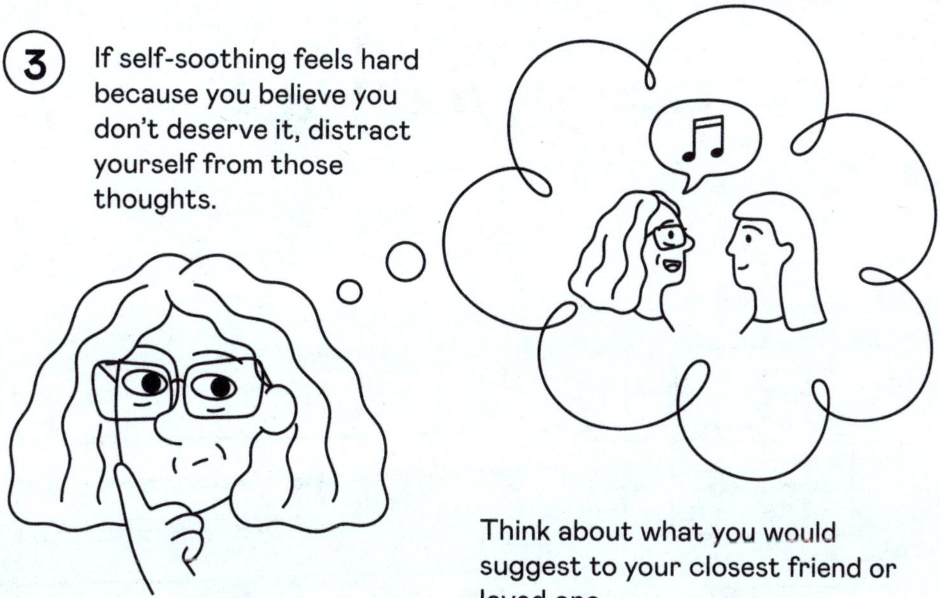

Think about what you would suggest to your closest friend or loved one.

4. Make a "self-soothe toolkit."

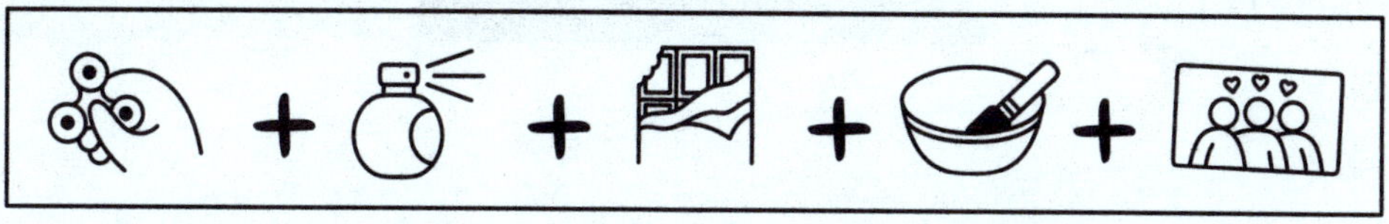

Use a shoebox, dopp kit, tote bag, or something similar, and put several **Self-Soothe** items inside.

Bring out that **self-soothe** toolkit in times of stress or crisis.

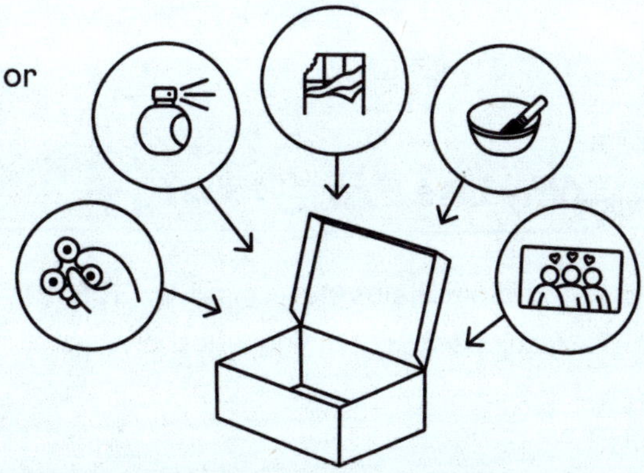

Consider having a toolkit for different contexts:

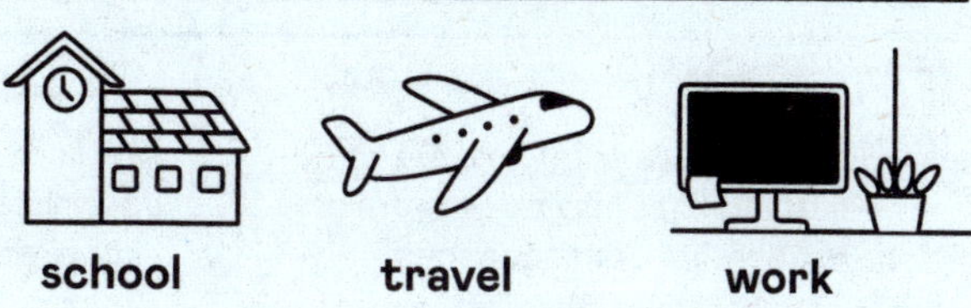

When Self-Soothe isn't effective, practice these skills:
PROBLEM SOLVING · RADICAL ACCEPTANCE

PROS/CONS

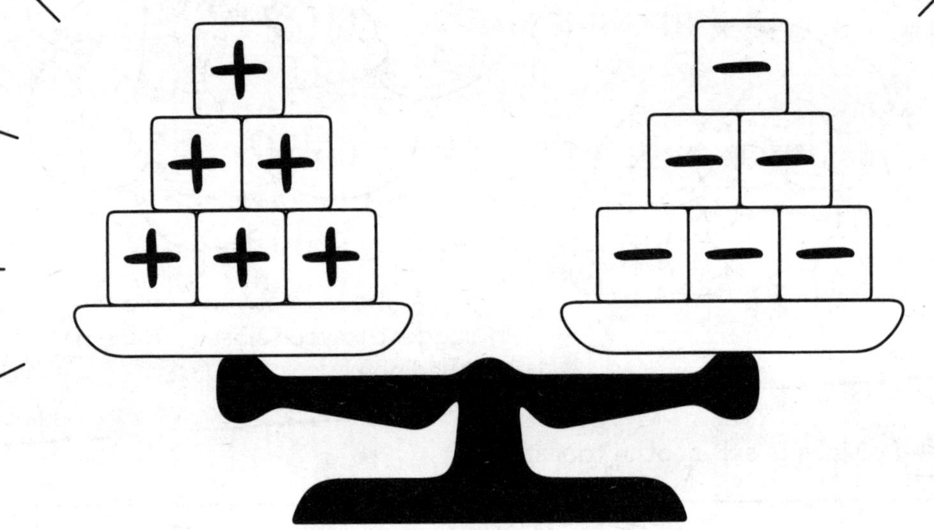

Why Use Pros/Cons?

Pros/Cons helps determine the effective course of action. It can be useful specifically for deciding whether to give in to crisis urges or ride them out.

When to Use Pros/Cons

☑ **Use when:**

- You are experiencing an urge to do something that may be harmful or have negative consequences.
- You are stuck making a decision between two options.

☒ **Do NOT use when:**

You are just trying to give yourself permission to do something that you know will be an ineffective behavior. (This is an unmindful Pros/Cons!)

PROS/CONS is a system to help you decide between two courses of action. In a comprehensive, Wise Mind way, you list the pros and cons of Action 1 and the pros and cons of Action 2. In this way, you create a 2×2 grid (see the next page). In DBT, we often use Pros/Cons to determine whether we should act on an urge or resist an urge.

For example, maybe your "go to" response to stress is to eat a lot of high-sugar, high-fat foods. You could do a Pros/Cons evaluation where you write out the Pros/Cons of eating a lot of those foods in response to stress *and* the Pros/Cons of not eating those foods in response to stress and doing some alternative. Or maybe you have been offered a new job and you're not sure if you should take it. You could write out the Pros/Cons of taking the job *and* the Pros/Cons of not taking the job/staying in your current job. You can also use your different states of mind to complete it (What does Emotion Mind tell you? What does Reasonable Mind say? What would Wise Mind do?)

By taking such a thorough approach to the issue, you may find that you generate Pros/Cons that surprise you. Or you discover why it's been so hard to change a behavior because you see all that the behavior is doing for you in the short-term. It's also important to know that the "answer" does not necessarily lie within the box that has the most items. Instead, once you have a completed Pros/Cons grid, take it all in and use your Wise Mind to determine the effective course of action.

How to Know If Pros/Cons Is Working

Pros/Cons is effective if you identify one course of action as having more significant pros and less significant cons than another course of action and you use that to guide your choice.

How to: Pros/Cons

1 Use **Pros/Cons** when trying to decide a course of action and access **Wise Mind.**

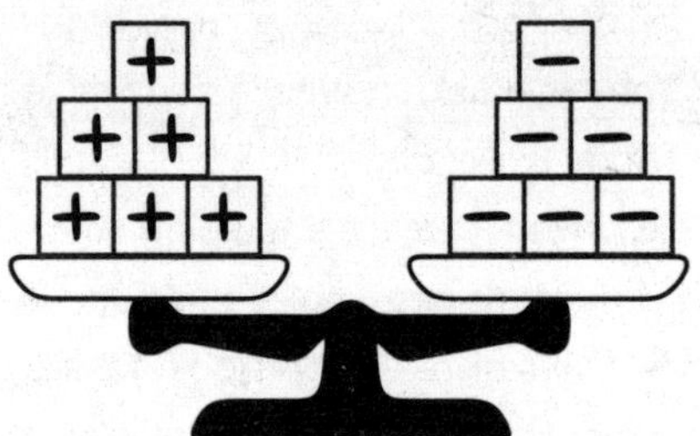

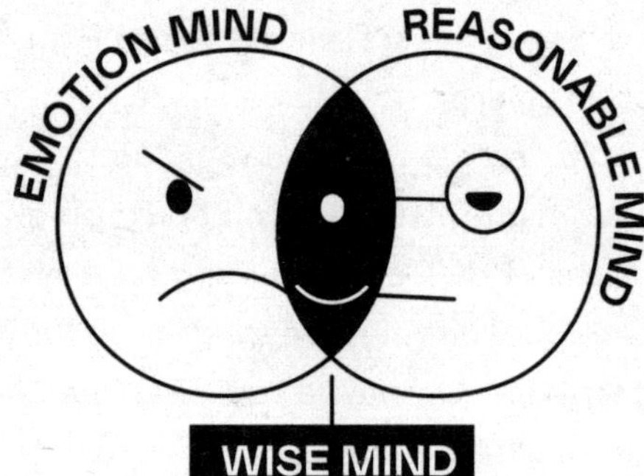

Pros/Cons can be especially helpful when you have an intense urge to do something problematic.

Even taking the time to write a **Pros/Cons** can help you ride out the urge for a few minutes and get you into a better place.

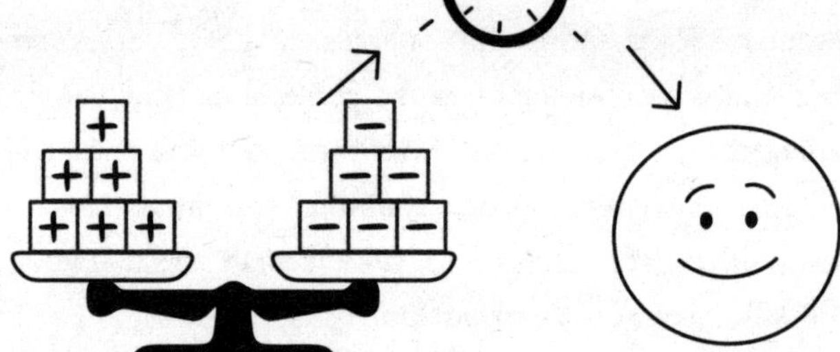

2 Draw a grid.

	+ *Pros*	− *Cons*
Action 1 *Acting on Urge*		
Action 2 *Resisting Urge*		

3. Accessing your different states of mind (**Emotion Mind**, **Reasonable Mind**, **Wise Mind**), list all **Pros and Cons** you can think of. Don't censor.

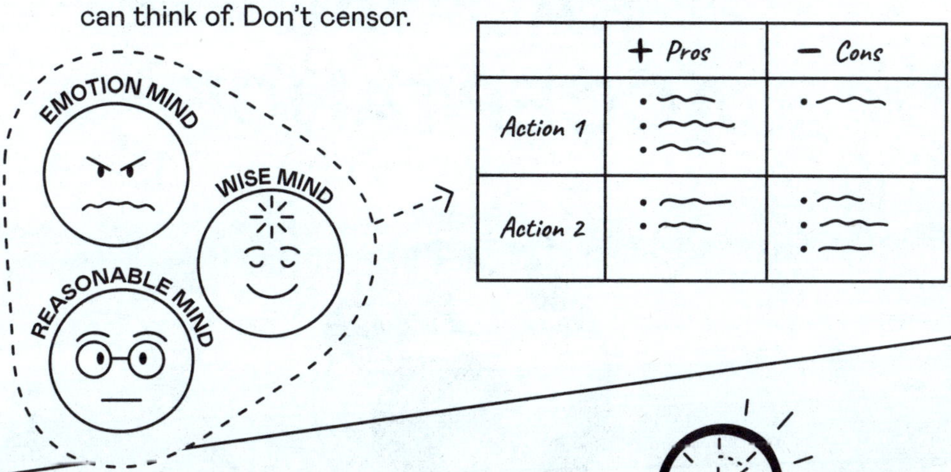

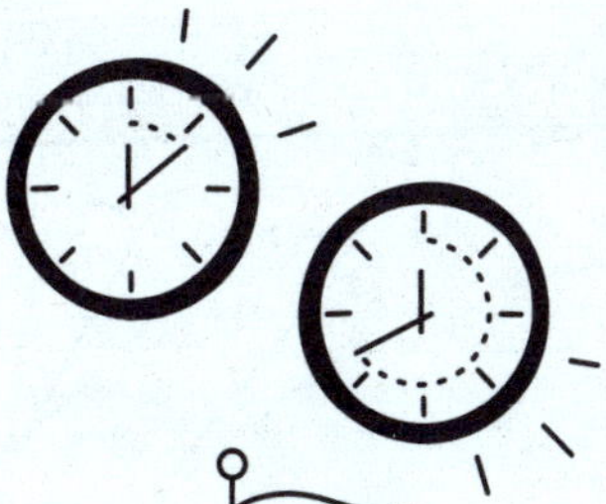

EMOTION MIND

WISE MIND

REASONABLE MIND

	+ Pros	− Cons
Action 1	• ~~ • ~~ • ~~	• ~~
Action 2	• ~~ • ~~	• ~~ • ~~ • ~~

4. Reflect on each quadrant, the number of items listed, the consequences of each item, and how those consequences impact your long-term goals.

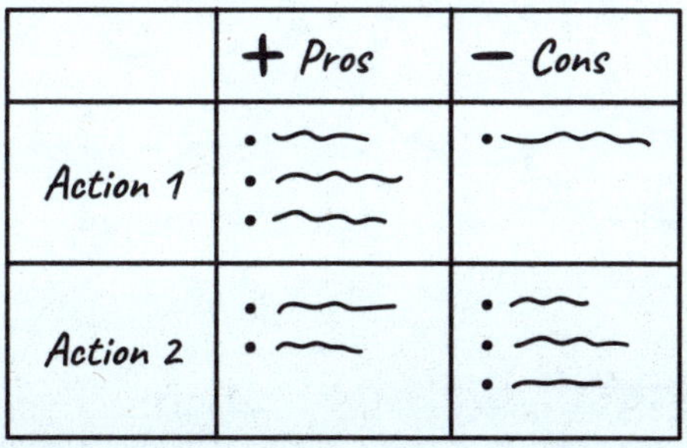

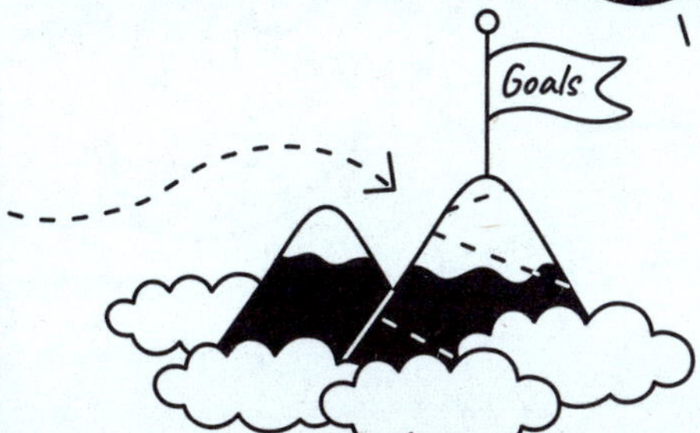

	+ Pros	− Cons
Action 1	• ~~ • ~~ • ~~	• ~~
Action 2	• ~~ • ~~	• ~~ • ~~ • ~~

Goals

Keep in mind: You are *not* looking for the quadrant with the most items listed. Sometimes there is one item listed, but that item is super important.

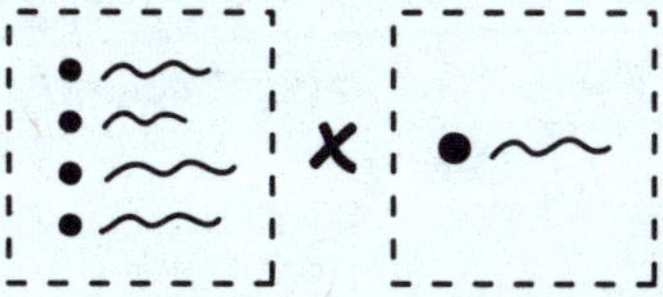

5. You can use the **Pros/Cons** list to make a decision in the moment or you can refer to a completed **Pros/Cons** in more difficult moments.

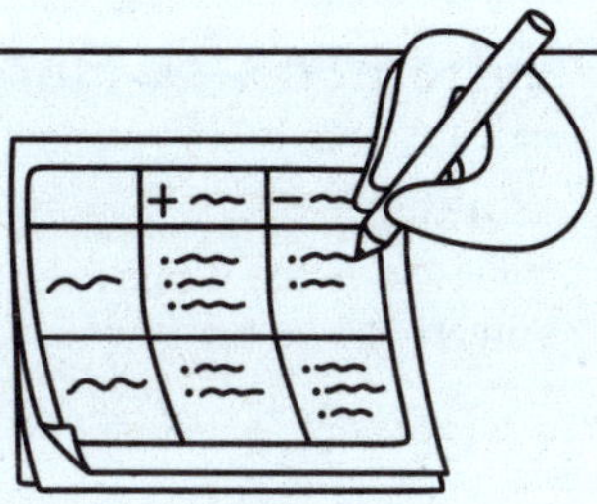

When Pros/Cons isn't effective, practice these skills:

TIP · DISTRACT · IMPROVE · SELF-SOOTHE

RADICAL ACCEPTANCE

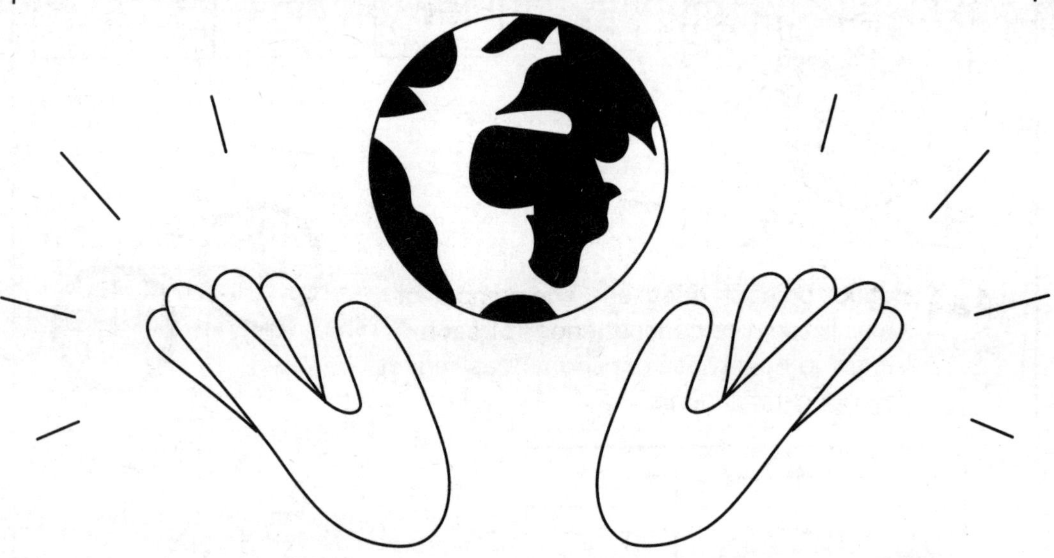

Why Use Radical Acceptance?

The skill of Radical Acceptance helps us accept reality and thereby reduce our suffering.

When to Use Radical Acceptance

☑ **Use when:**

Your life or the world is not exactly how you want it to be, that is, most of the time!

☒ **Do NOT use when:**

You are too dysregulated by the situation to think straight. In those moments, practicing other skills to become more regulated will put you in a better position to practice Radical Acceptance.

RADICAL ACCEPTANCE is a reality acceptance distress tolerance skill. It is the practice of accepting this moment and this reality exactly as it is, no matter how much you wish it were different or how much you hate it. To practice Radical Acceptance, you can recognize and accept that this moment couldn't be any other way, given the billions and billions of events that have led up to it. In other words, this moment is caused. You may not know, like, or approve of the causes, but they have created the reality of this moment. Another way to practice this skill is to take a deep breath and say something to yourself like "everything is as it should be" or "I accept this moment exactly as it is." The "radical" part of Radical Acceptance means practicing it with mind, body, and soul—all the way, completely.

Radical Acceptance also means fully accepting yourself, your views, your feelings, and your opinions. Just like the moment itself, your feelings about the moment are caused, too. Even if you don't know what the causes are, you can trust that there are experiences, including biological ones that you can't see, that have shaped you.

Radical Acceptance does *not* mean that you must like or approve of the situation; instead, it is the practice of accepting that the moment could not be otherwise. This can be a profound shift in how you experience your life! Radical Acceptance involves turning your mind away from rejecting reality ("it shouldn't be this way"), which usually creates more suffering. Instead, you notice when you are rejecting reality and then move toward accepting the reality with your mind and body.

Radical acceptance will not eliminate pain from your life—pain is inevitable and part of being human. However, practicing Radical Acceptance will help reduce your suffering. So often we add to our pain by resisting reality. In addition, accepting reality exactly as it is often helps us be in a better place to make changes. In that sense, Radical Acceptance is a precursor to change.

How to Know If Radical Acceptance Is Working

Radical Acceptance is a skill that requires a lot of practice and effort. Over time, if you stop running away from reality, you will become more effective, and therefore more likely to reach your goals, enact positive changes, and make the next moments ones that are easier to accept.

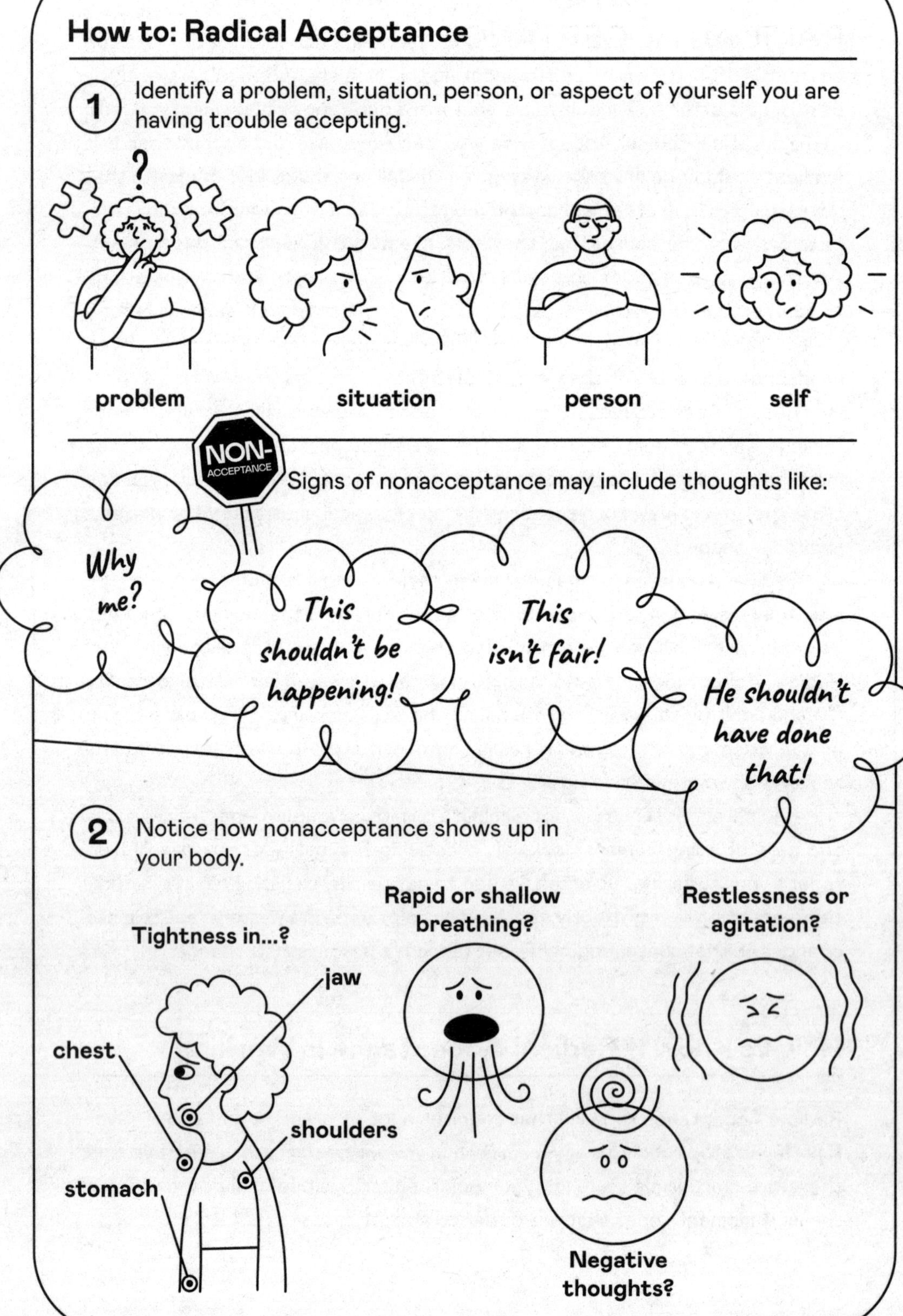
How to: Radical Acceptance
1 Identify a problem, situation, person, or aspect of yourself you are having trouble accepting.
?
problem
situation
person
self
NON-
ACCEPTANCE
Signs of nonacceptance may include thoughts like:
Why me?
This shouldn't be happening!
This isn't fair!
He shouldn't have done that!
2 Notice how nonacceptance shows up in your body.
Tightness in...?
jaw
chest
shoulders
stomach
Rapid or shallow breathing?
Restlessness or agitation?
Negative thoughts?

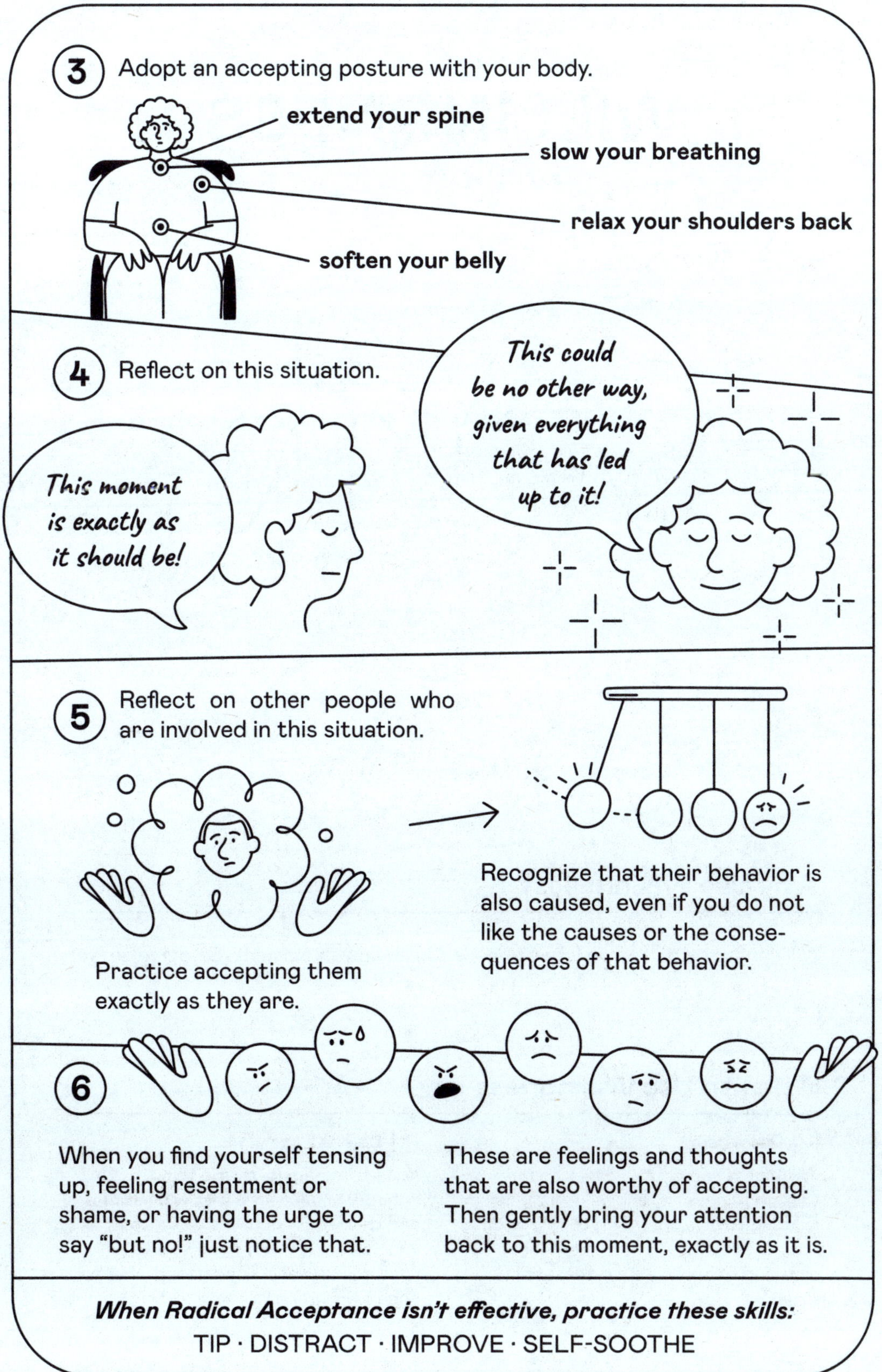
3
Adopt an accepting posture with your body.
extend your spine
slow your breathing
relax your shoulders back
soften your belly
4
Reflect on this situation.
This moment is exactly as it should be!
This could be no other way, given everything that has led up to it!
5
Reflect on other people who are involved in this situation.
Practice accepting them exactly as they are.
Recognize that their behavior is also caused, even if you do not like the causes or the consequences of that behavior.
6
When you find yourself tensing up, feeling resentment or shame, or having the urge to say "but no!" just notice that.
These are feelings and thoughts that are also worthy of accepting. Then gently bring your attention back to this moment, exactly as it is.
When Radical Acceptance isn't effective, practice these skills:
TIP · DISTRACT · IMPROVE · SELF-SOOTHE

WILLINGNESS

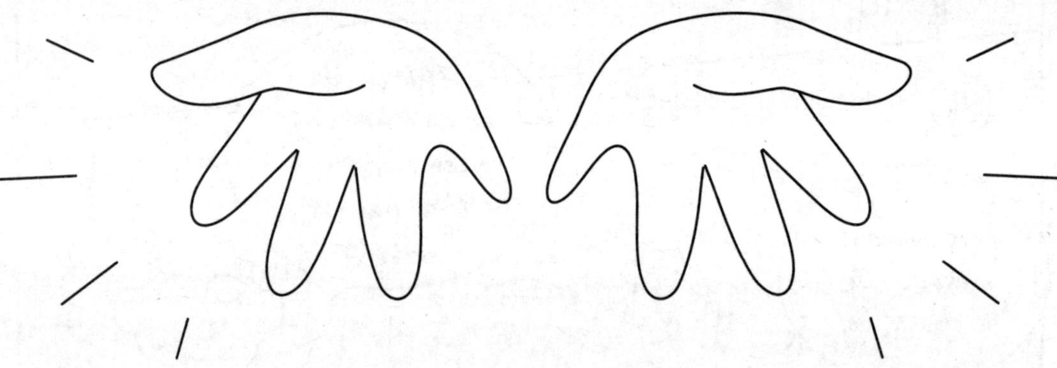

Why Use Willingness?

Willingness helps you do what's needed in any given moment. By doing so, you learn to act with awareness and less effort.

When to Use Willingness

☑ **Use when:**

Willfulness shows up. Some clues that willfulness has shown up include wanting to give up, trying to refuse or deny the reality of the moment, and/or trying to control everything about a situation.

☒ **Do NOT use when:**

You are engaging (or are tempted to engage) in behaviors that are harmful and that are contrary to your goals and values. You may need to clarify your goals to help understand what to engage in willingly.

WILLINGNESS refers to approaching any situation with an attitude of "yes" rather than "no"—to participate fully in life, no matter what it hands you. It is a reality acceptance distress tolerance skill.

Willingness is closely related to the mindfulness skill of Effectively: being willing to do what is needed in this one moment rather than refusing or avoiding. It is also closely related to the skill of Radical Acceptance because Willingness usually coincides with accepting the moment exactly as it is. In contrast, when we are willful, we are trying to shape reality to our preferences. (Spoiler alert: That doesn't work! It's like throwing a tantrum rather than accepting consequences gracefully.)

Willingness involves first noticing if you are being willful (that is, rejecting reality). If so, you have arrived at a fork in the road and have to make a choice. Do you want to stay on the path of willfulness even if that means not getting what you want or experiencing other negative consequences? Or do you want to turn your mind toward the path of willingness? If so, take the first step down the willingness path by adopting a willing posture (see next page) and finding a willing course of action. You may have to engage in this process many, many times if the situation is challenging or if you're stuck in a rut of willfulness. It will get easier with practice!

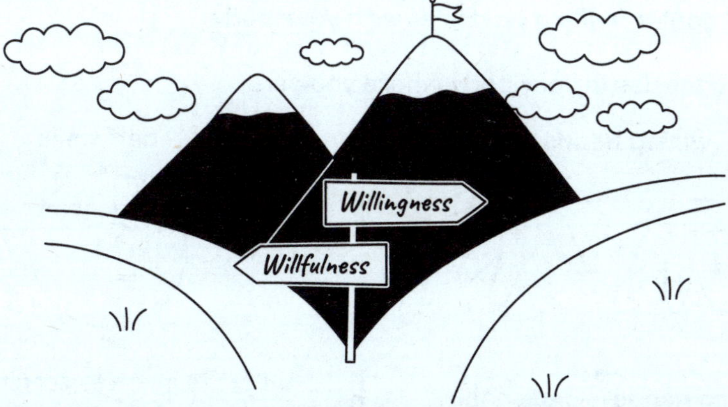

How to Know If Willingness Is Working

Willingness is often associated with feeling unstuck. Along with the skill of Effectively, it usually helps move you forward on a problem. Although willingness can be challenging to practice, when you become more skilled at it, willingness actually takes less effort and energy than being willful does.

How to: Willingness

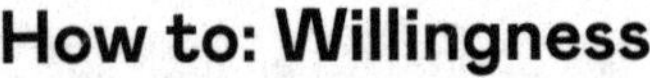

1. Notice when you're experiencing willfulness. Usually this takes the form of:

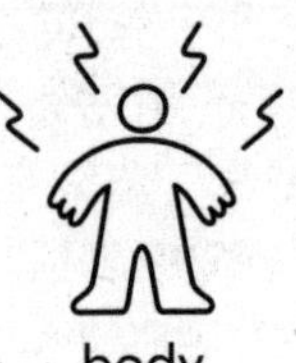

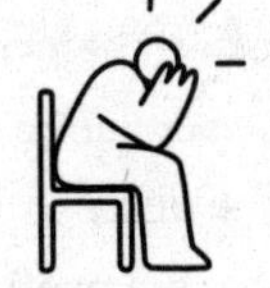

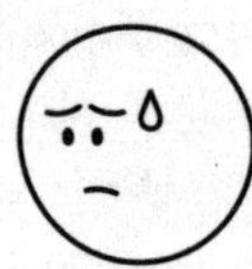

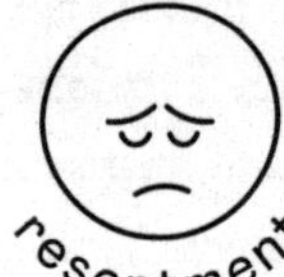

And may include thoughts like:

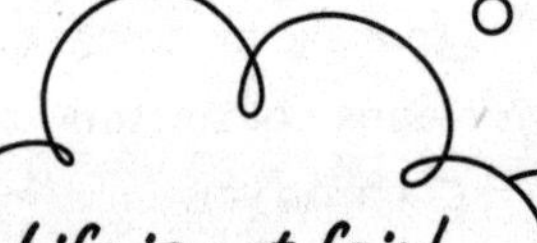

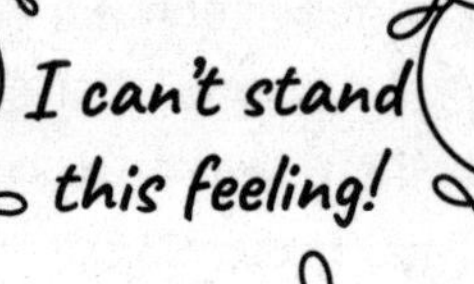

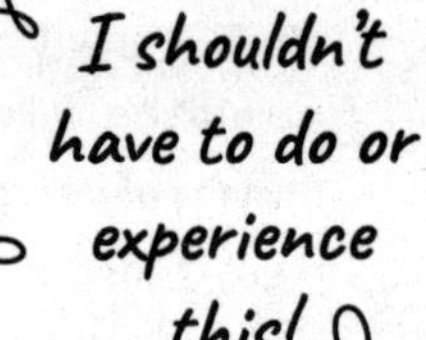

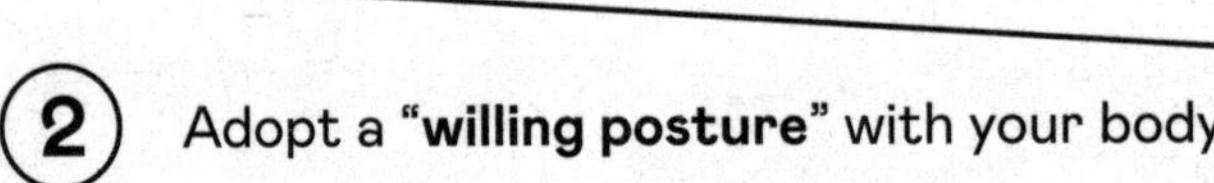

2. Adopt a **"willing posture"** with your body:

Relax the tension in your body where you can.

willing hands

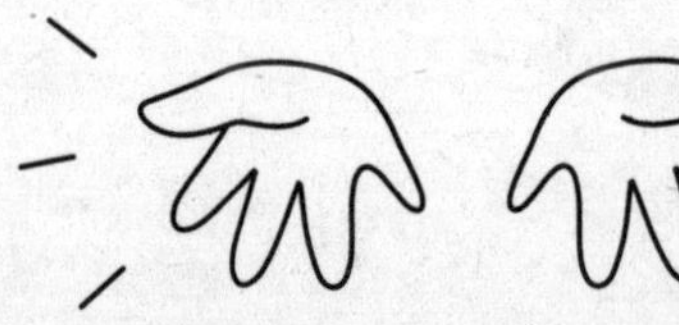

Willing hands is unclenching your hands and, if sitting, resting them on your lap with the palms face up.

half smile

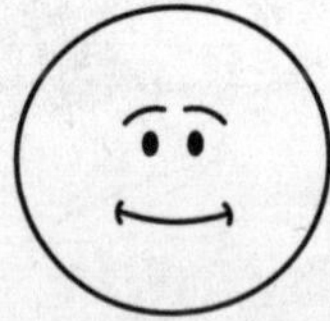

Half smile involves turning up the corners of your mouth so that you are smiling a little bit, but not so much that it feels forced or fake.

These changes to your body indicate to your brain that you are more open and willing to accept your reality.

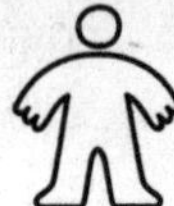

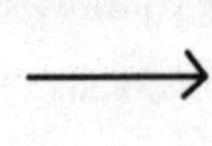

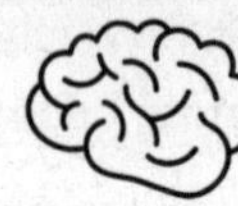

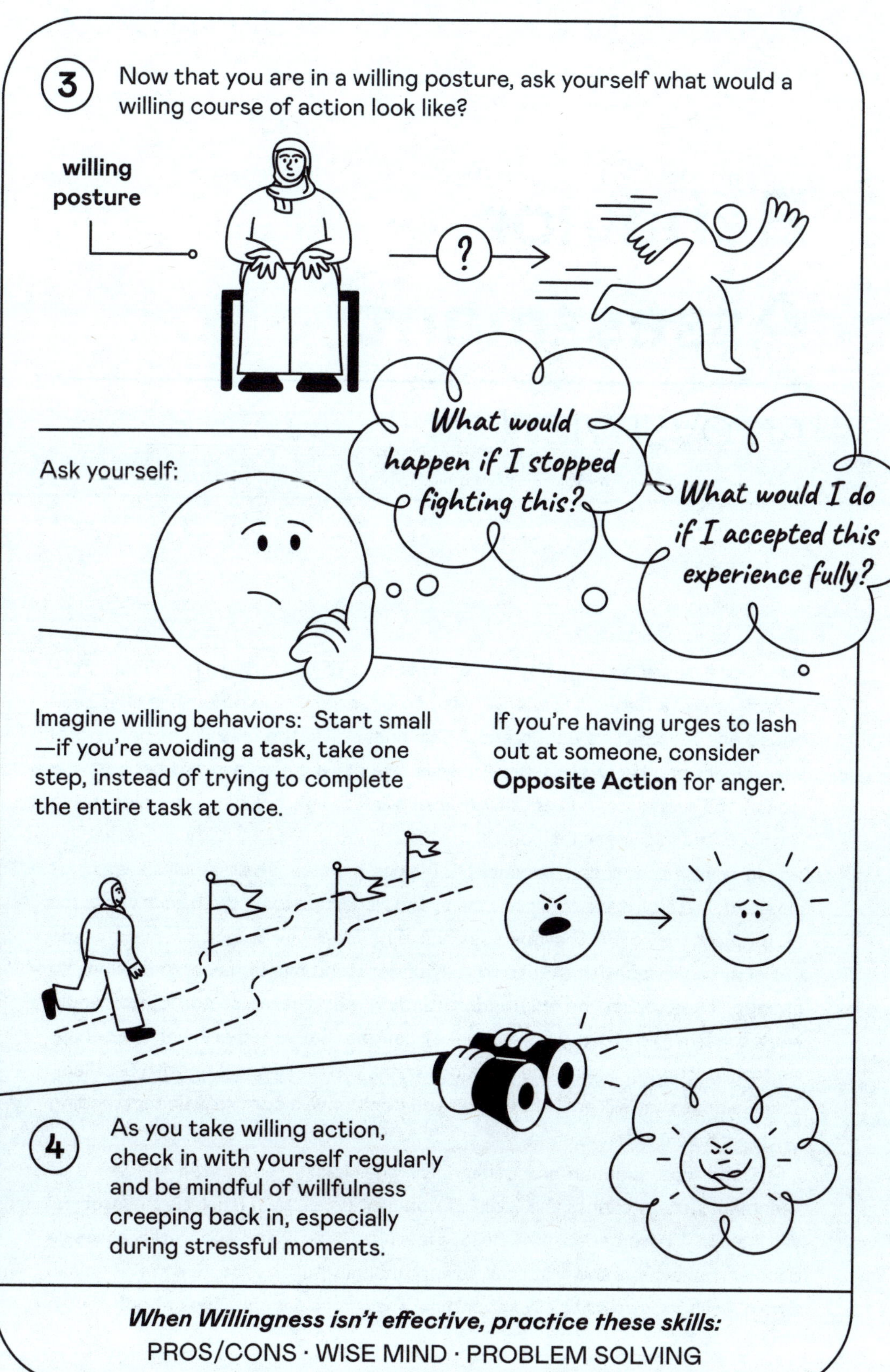
3
Now that you are in a willing posture, ask yourself what would a willing course of action look like?
willing posture
?
Ask yourself:
What would happen if I stopped fighting this?
What would I do if I accepted this experience fully?
Imagine willing behaviors: Start small —if you're avoiding a task, take one step, instead of trying to complete the entire task at once.
If you're having urges to lash out at someone, consider **Opposite Action** for anger.
4
As you take willing action, check in with yourself regularly and be mindful of willfulness creeping back in, especially during stressful moments.
When Willingness isn't effective, practice these skills:
PROS/CONS · WISE MIND · PROBLEM SOLVING

Behavior Assessment

AN OVERVIEW

Behavior assessment is the systematic process of gathering all relevant information about a behavior that we wish to change, including events that preceded and followed its occurrence. Our final skill is the method of behavioral assessment used in DBT: Chain Analysis. We call it *chain* analysis because we look at the sequence of events from link to link to link, noticing how everything is connected in a linear fashion.

In Marsha Linehan's original DBT skills manual, Chain Analysis was not included. Instead, it was only taught to DBT therapists as the primary tool for assessing behavior in therapy sessions. The idea was that therapists would use chain analyses with clients to fully understand the behavior they want to change. Then, based on this understanding, the therapist and client would work together to identify how to make changes that would prevent the behavior from occurring again. The thinking is that you can't come up with problem-solving ideas that will actually work if you don't have a complete understanding of the problem behavior first.

Over time, Linehan and other DBT therapists recognized the value of teaching therapy clients the "skill" of conducting a Chain Analysis themselves. We include it here because we believe learning to fully and accurately assess a problem behavior is the first step toward meaningful change. (One of us thinks Chain Analysis is so critically important, she wrote a whole book about it!)

To change a behavior in a sustained way, we must understand the causes of the behavior and the consequences that are helping keep the behavior around. As we analyze a behavior over time through multiple chain analyses, we can spot recurring patterns, giving us valuable insights into which skills are best suited for changing that behavior. With practice, we also become more mindful of our own behavioral patterns and the sequence of events that contribute to them. This can be especially helpful if we tend to forget, or block out, painful details of our experiences. Although this mental avoidance makes sense in the moment because it distracts us from shame and guilt, it prevents us from making meaningful changes that can stop the behavior from occurring again.

It is important to note that behavior assessment alone is not sufficient for behavior change to occur. Change will require the implementation of solutions, like other skills found in this book.

Often, it can be difficult to identify exactly what happened leading up to a problem behavior, making a Chain Analysis ineffective. In that case, you can use other skills to learn to be more mindful of a sequence of events as it occurs. For example, you could use the PLEASE skills to address vulnerability factors, Problem Solving to address the Prompting Event, or Nonjudgmentally to address your thoughts and interpretations. There are so many options available to you now! This will help you be more skillful with Chain Analysis in the future.

CHAIN ANALYSIS

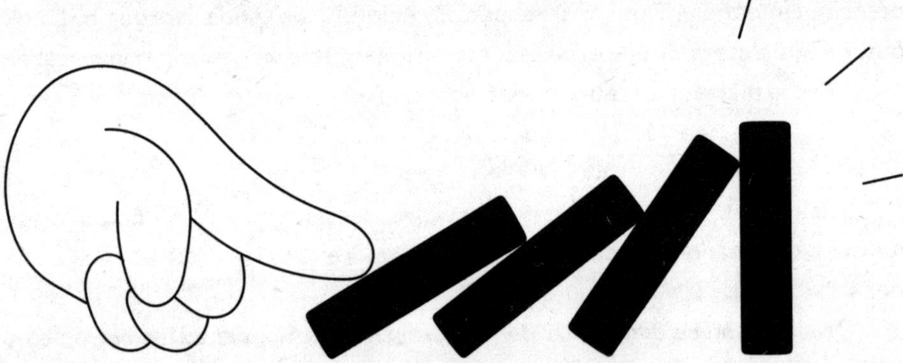

Why Use Chain Analysis?

Chain Analysis helps you understand a behavior in context so that you can be most successful at changing it.

When to Use Chain Analysis

☑ **Use when:**

- You want to understand why you engage in a particular behavior (and/or what function it serves for you).
- You want to change a behavior in a sustained way.

☒ **Do NOT use when:**

You're not interested in changing the behavior.

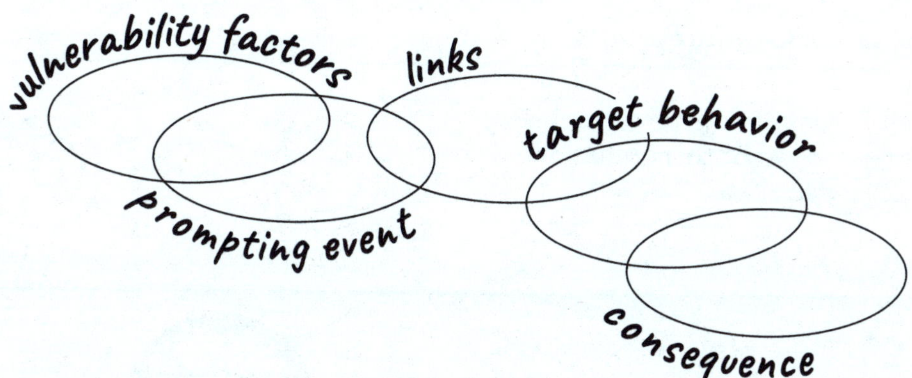

CHAIN ANALYSIS is a method for assessing a specific instance of a behavior. That means getting to know a behavior very well: what led up to its occurrence and what its consequences were.

Chain Analysis has five components:

1. The target behavior: This is the behavior that you want to change.
2. The prompting event: This is the event that set off the chain leading to the target behavior. If the prompting event hadn't occurred, then you likely would not have engaged in the target behavior.
3. Vulnerability factors: These include anything that makes you vulnerable to the prompting event in that instant.
4. Links: These links describe what happened between the prompting event and the target behavior. Links can be your behaviors, another person's behaviors, events, or your thoughts, emotions, and bodily sensations.
5. Consequences: Consequences refers to what happened following the problem behavior. There are two types of consequences: short term and long term. In Chain Analysis, you often focus more on the immediate, or short-term, consequences because they tend to have far more impact on the likelihood of the behavior occurring again.

How to Know If Chain Analysis Is Working

As an assessment tool, Chain Analysis is working when it helps you understand your behavior more fully so that you can identify potential effective solutions.

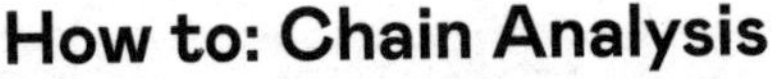

How to: Chain Analysis

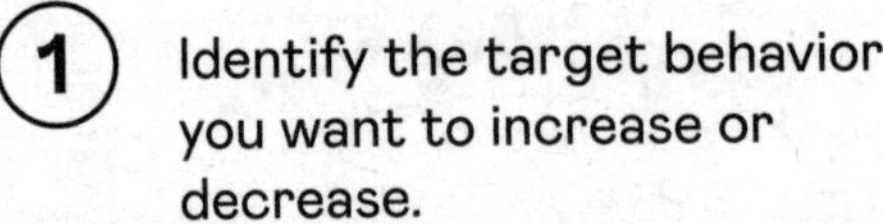

1 Identify the target behavior you want to increase or decrease.

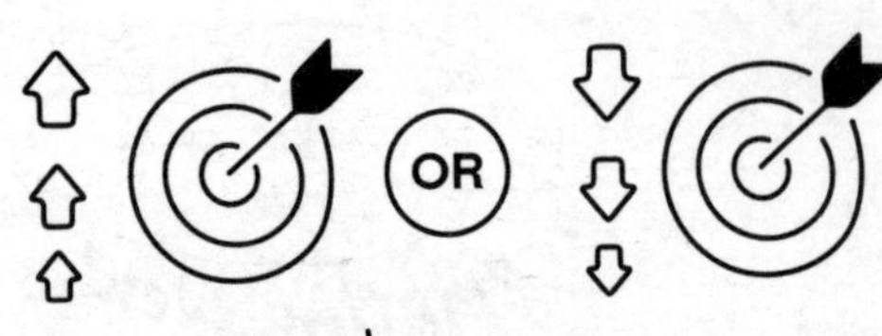

2 Think of a specific instance of this behavior.

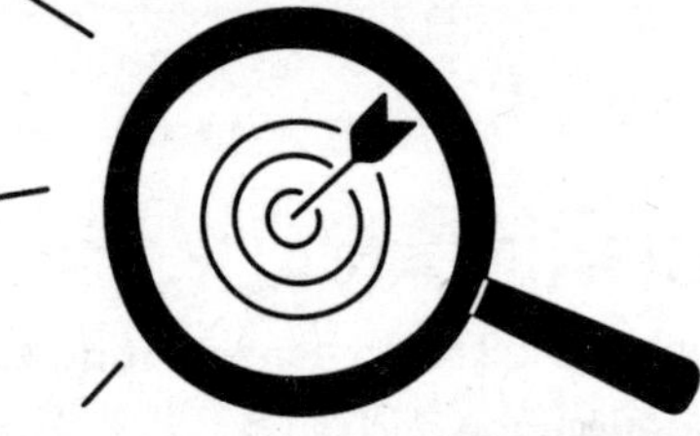

Use this instance to examine how to change the behavior.

This instance could be the most recent or the most intense form of the behavior.

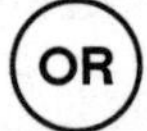

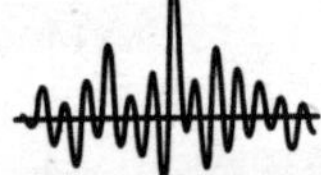

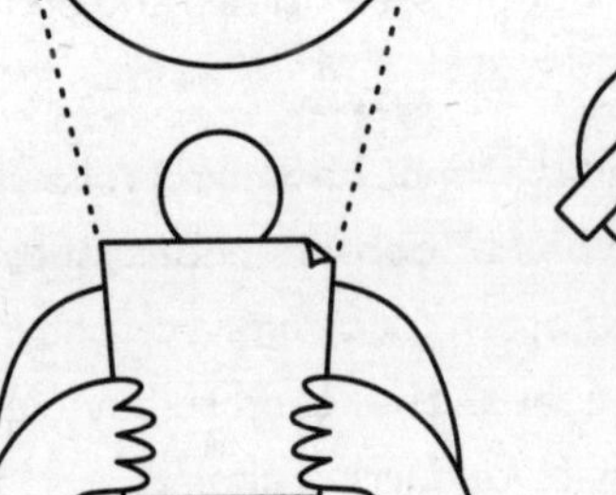

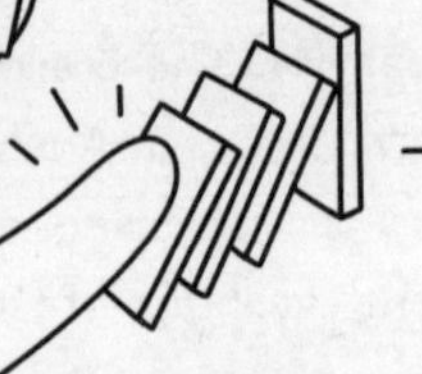

3 Identify the prompting event that set off the chain leading to the target behavior. It's like the first domino to fall.

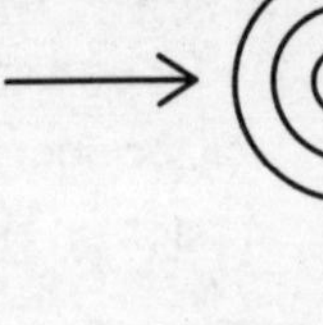

Describe the behavior very specifically as though you are writing a script and need the reader to "see" the behavior clearly.

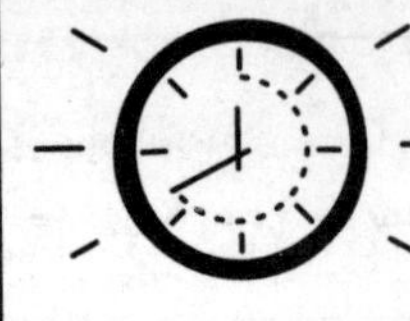

A typical prompting event occurs within a few hours or less of the target behavior.

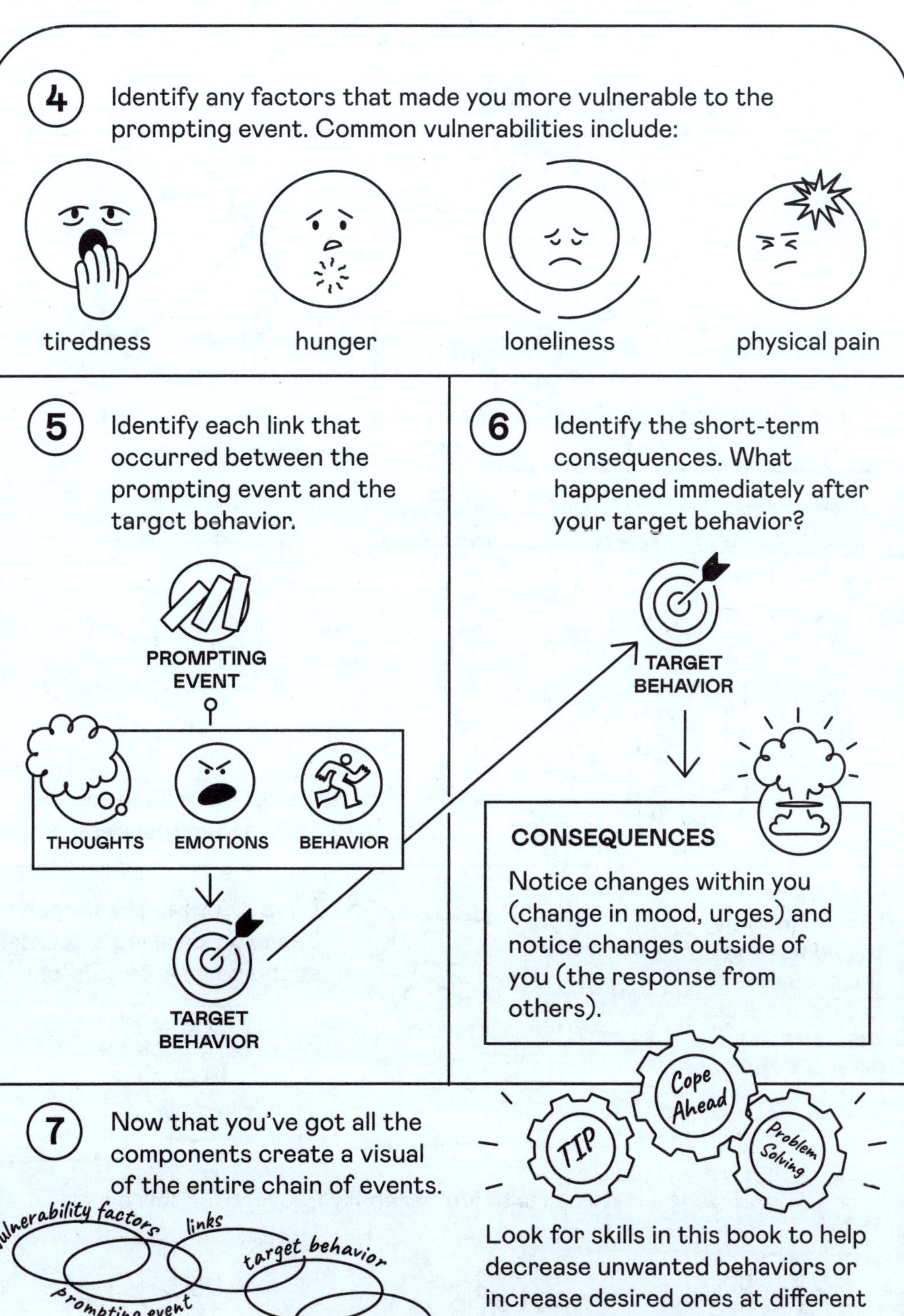

4 Identify any factors that made you more vulnerable to the prompting event. Common vulnerabilities include: tiredness, hunger, loneliness, physical pain

5 Identify each link that occurred between the prompting event and the target behavior.

6 Identify the short-term consequences. What happened immediately after your target behavior?

CONSEQUENCES

Notice changes within you (change in mood, urges) and notice changes outside of you (the response from others).

7 Now that you've got all the components create a visual of the entire chain of events.

Look for skills in this book to help decrease unwanted behaviors or increase desired ones at different points in the chain.

When Chain Analysis isn't effective, practice these skills:
OBSERVE · DESCRIBE

In Practice: Chain Analysis

Meet Dave.

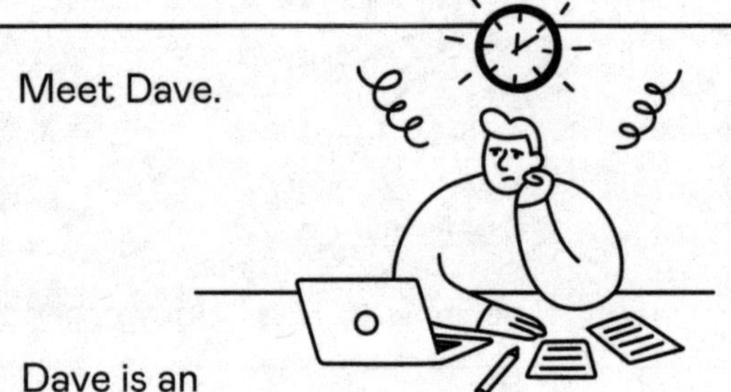

Dave is an overworked graphic designer who's been burning the candle at both ends.

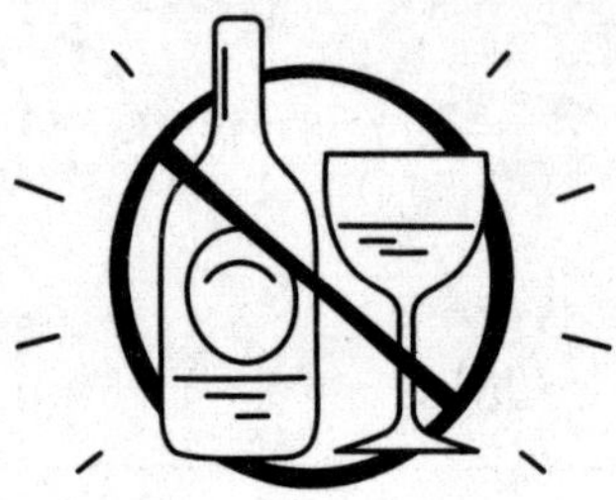

Dave has been sober for almost two years.

After a particularly rough week at work, Dave went to a birthday party and ended up drinking.

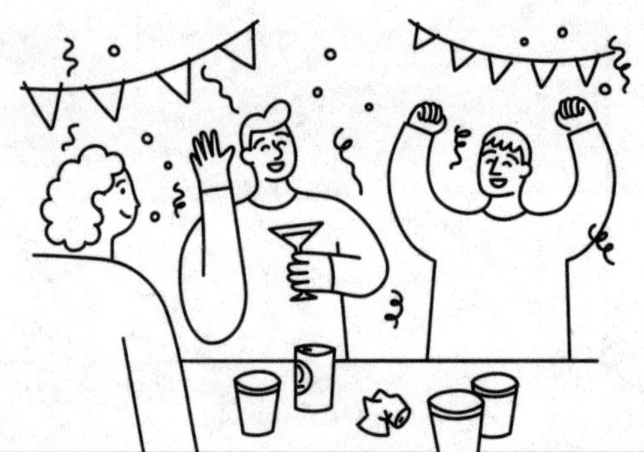

He felt out of control and now feels deeply ashamed and hopeless.

Dave uses **Chain Analysis** to understand the sequence of events so he can learn to make different choices next time.

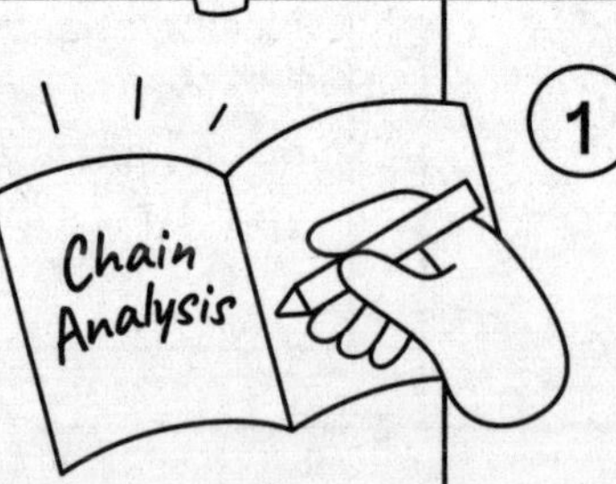

1 Dave identifies the **target behavior**: drinking a cocktail at the party around 10pm.

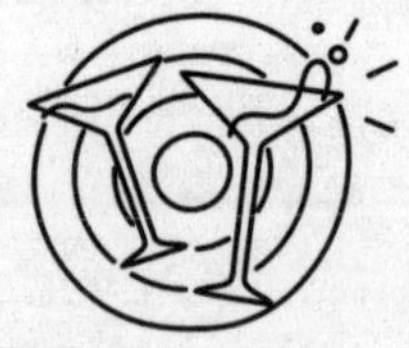

3 Dave identifies three major **Vulnerabilty Factors** for this event:

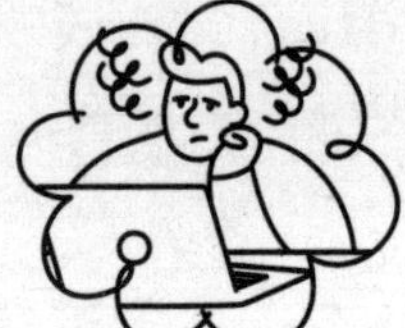

work stress

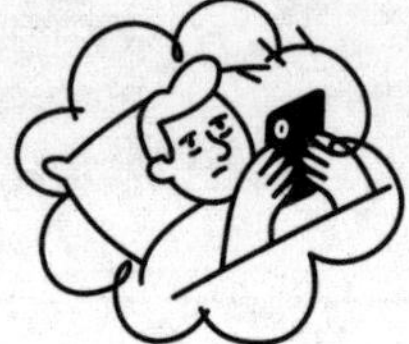

fatigue

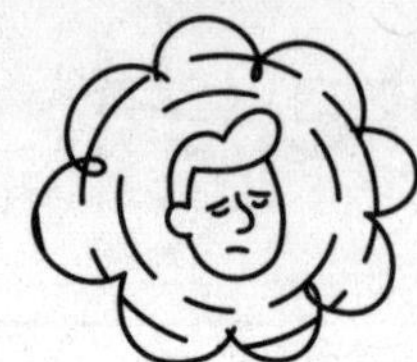

loneliness

(4) Dave identifies the **prompting event**:

A cutie at the bar offered to get him a drink.

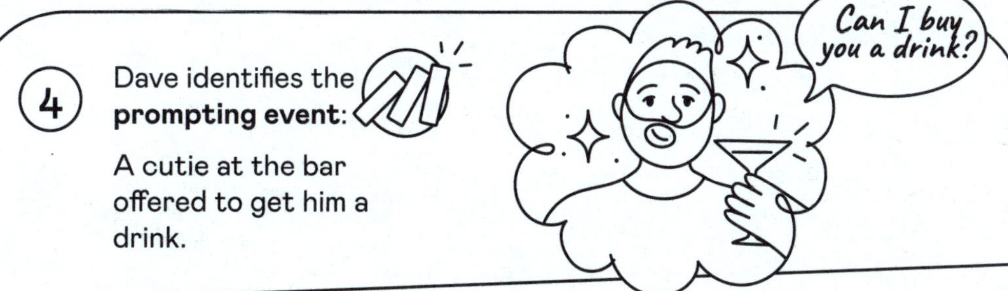

(5) Dave traces the links leading to his target behavior, noticing his thoughts, feelings, and actions along the way.

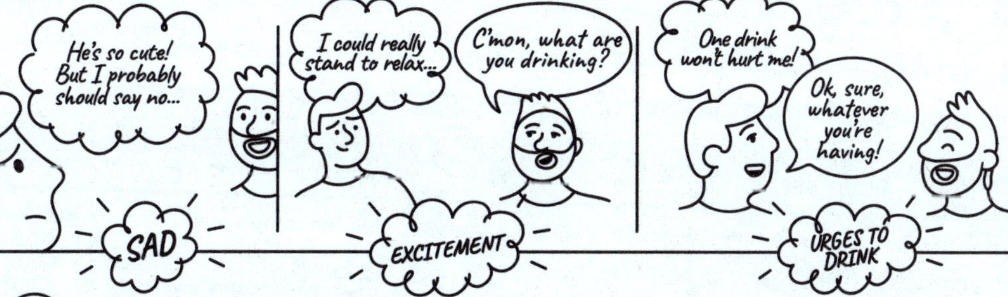

(6) Dave then explores the short-term and long-term consequences.

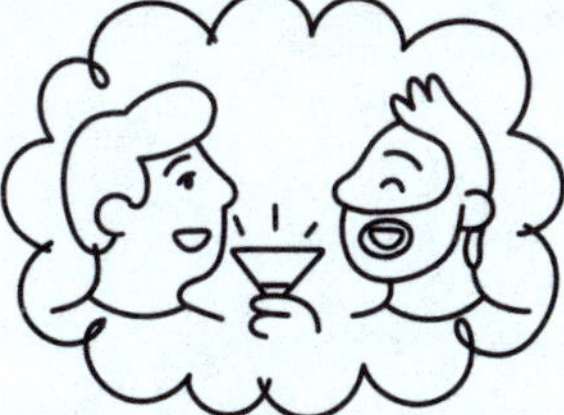

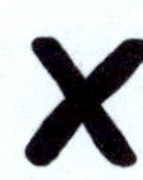

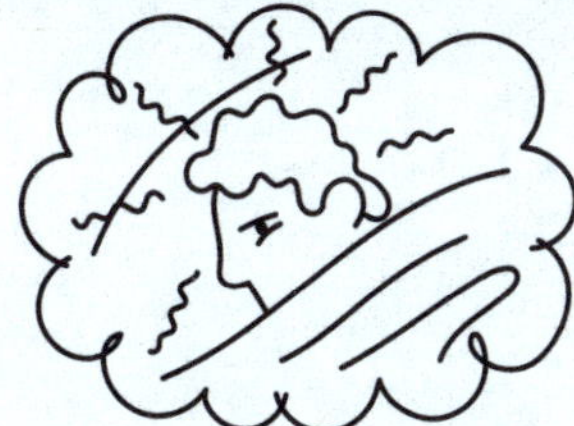

In the short-term, Dave found that the alcohol made him feel more confident and willing to talk to the cute guy. He ended up having two more drinks over the next two hours.

In the long-term, Dave slept poorly that night and woke up with a headache. He feels intense shame and guilt about his lapse and worries that he set himself up to continue to have a drinking problem.

(7) With insights from **Chain Analysis**, Dave plans to use skills like **PLEASE**, **DEAR MAN**, **Pros/Cons** and **Self-Soothe** to make healthier choices at future parties.

List of Skills:

- PLEASE: Reduce vulnerability (e.g., manage stress, nap before the party).
- DEAR MAN: Firmly say no to drinks even when he has urges to say "yes."
- Pros/Cons: Write out a pros/cons list for drinking.
- Self-Soothe: Relax after work with a warm bath and favorite music.

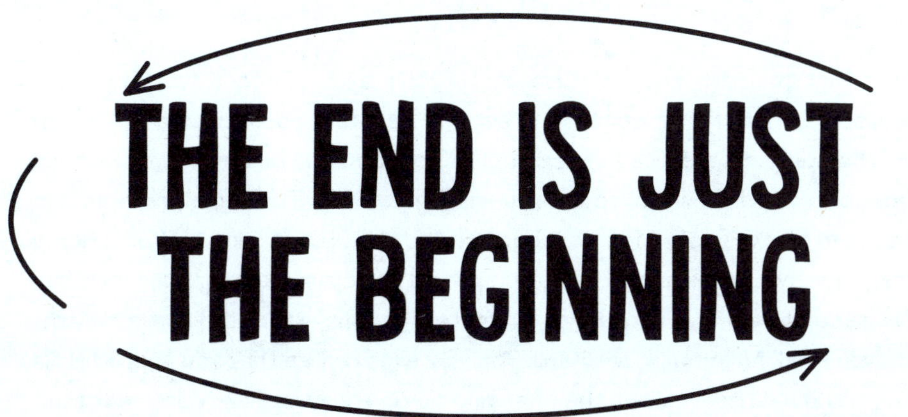

THE END IS JUST THE BEGINNING

You've made it! You've now learned dozens of skills to help you navigate life more effectively. How does it feel? We hope you feel more empowered and ready to take on whatever life throws your way.

In this final section, we describe ways to integrate these skills throughout your day for a more balanced and effective life. In addition to using these skills in response to difficult moments, you can also use them in proactive and consistent ways every day. Our goal is to help you build a life worth living, not just one of putting out fires as they arise, so you can approach challenges with a sense of pride and mastery.

There are two takeaway points in this section.

1. Practice these skills as often as possible.
2. Don't only use these skills in response to crises and challenging moments. Instead, practice some of these skills on a regular basis to reduce your vulnerability to crises and to create more balance in your life.

Practice these skills as often as possible. Use them proactively and not just in response to crises and challenging moments.

Here we walk you through some tips for helping make this happen.

In the introduction to this book, we used the analogy of traveling to a foreign country and not knowing the language. We discussed how overcoming that deficit starts with learning one word at a time. Anybody who has learned another language as an adult knows that the early stages of learning involve a lot of effort: word-by-word translations, practicing common greetings, learning to both speak and listen. The goal is to achieve fluency, that is, to ultimately communicate without translating word by word, to communicate naturally. The same principle can be applied to skills use. After you acquire the skills by learning and practicing a few times, you will want to keep using them in ways that, over time, become more second nature and intuitive. Ultimately, you may start to use them without even thinking about it too hard. You may even realize that you applied skills *after* you used them rather than needing to do every skill with premeditated intention. That's amazing when it happens!

Practice Makes (Near) Perfect

Of course, dialectically, we know nothing is perfect and conflict-free. As one of Shireen's favorite lines from her favorite movie, *The Princess Bride,** goes: "Life is pain, Highness. Anyone who says differently is selling something." Practicing these skills will not take away all your pain and struggle. Nor do we want them to! For example, no amount of skills use will take away the pain of losing a loved one. However, as you become more skillful in response to difficult moments in your life, you may find that you cope with pain in ways that feel less impulsive and more consistent with your values. You may also find that you learn the fundamentals of painful experiences: that they won't last forever, that they may teach you something about yourself and your values, and that they are universal.

Practicing skills is like any new habit. It may take a while for it to become second nature, and at first you might have difficulty even remembering that these skills exist! So the first step might be to ask yourself how you can remember to practice these skills on a regular basis. Here are some ideas to consider; try them and choose what works for you.

- Set alarms on your phone, put sticky notes around your home, or send yourself reminders.
- Create some accountability to another person—like a friend or family

*Incidentally, watching *The Princess Bride* would be a great Distract or Self-Soothe if it's a repeat comfort viewing!

member who can be your skills buddy. You both commit to practicing and checking in with each other every day.

- Complete what we call a "daily diary card" in DBT treatment. Part of that card includes the list of DBT skills, and clients indicate on the card which skills they practiced on any given day. Maybe you want to make your own version of a skills diary card—on paper or on a device—so that you can review them and indicate which ones you've practiced on any given day. It can look something like this:

SKILLS	M	T	W	T	F	S	S
MINDFULNESS	✓	✓	✓	✓	✓	✓	✓
RADICAL ACCEPTANCE					✓	✓	✓
ACCUMULATE POSITIVES (SHORT-TERM)	✓	✓	✓	✓	✓	✓	✓
ACCUMULATE POSITIVES (LONG-TERM)		✓	✓	✓	✓		
PLEASE	✓	✓		✓	✓		

When you practice, make sure to reward yourself in some way for doing the practice. This is a simple behavioral trick that increases the likelihood you'll practice more in the future. Maybe it's a metaphorical pat on the back and telling yourself sincerely, "Awesome job today. I'm killing it!" Maybe it's a small treat that you wouldn't ordinarily have: some chocolate or an extra episode of your favorite show. Remember to reward the *practice* of the skill, not whether the skill "worked." This is an especially important point for you perfectionists out there. In learning your language, that is, the skills, you are rewarding yourself for any practice, not perfect pronunciation or syntax. Rewarding yourself will help you stay more motivated to keep practicing.

Remember: Daily practice of the skills is the goal. It can be a 10-second mindfulness exercise of Observe or 30 minutes of preparing and delivering DEAR MAN GIVE FAST. And when you practice, give yourself the satisfaction of a check mark on your tracker and another small reward.

> *Aim for daily practice of the skills.*

Setting the Stage for a More Skillful Life

As you've likely noticed, some of the skills described in this book are situation specific. For example, you use the TIP skills when you are so distressed that you can't even think straight. You use Opposite Action when you want to change your experience of an emotion that doesn't fit the facts of the situation. You use DEAR MAN when you need to ask somebody for something. You can practice these skills at other times, of course, and doing so will make them easier to use when you really need them.

Other skills are not necessarily situation specific, and you would benefit from practicing them more regularly, whether you think you need them or not. We recommend practicing the mindfulness, PLEASE, ABC, and Radical Acceptance skills every day. We make this recommendation because the mindfulness skills can be incorporated into everything you do and provide the foundation for all the other skills. The PLEASE and ABC skills are about reducing your vulnerability to Emotion Mind and stress and require more consistent practice in order to have the maximum effect. And Radical Acceptance because . . . life.

Here are some tips for incorporating these skills into your daily life in simple ways:

Mindfulness skills (pages 16–41):

• Pause a few times throughout your day to identify what state of mind you're in. Are you in Reasonable Mind: focused on a task at hand without incorporating feelings or values? Are you in Emotion Mind: wanting to do whatever your emotion is telling you to do? Or are you in Wise Mind: integrating these two pieces and feeling a sense of centeredness in the process? If you're not in Wise Mind and that's causing problems for you, practice one of the Wise Mind exercises for a minute or two and notice its effects.

• Set a reminder or an alarm for different times of your day, and whenever it goes off, stop, pause, and practice Observe and Describe of this one moment. Or use that reminder to cue you to fully, and One-Mindfully, Participate in whatever task you're engaged in at this moment.

• When you notice irritation, jealousy, shame, or fear, see if you're adding any judgments to your experience. Try describing what you're reacting to in nonjudgmental terms. See if that changes anything about how you feel.

• When you find yourself in conflict with another person or fighting with yourself, ask whether you'd rather be right or effective. Think about what actions go along with being right and what actions go along with being effective. Do the actions that are in line with your goal.

PLEASE and ABC (pages 84–91):

• Remember to do something every day that gives you a sense of pleasure and joy. This is accumulating positives (A) in the short term.

• Take an action every day, no matter how small, that gets you closer to a more long-term goal. This is accumulating positives (A) in the long term.

• Similarly, take an action every day, no matter how small, that makes you feel a sense of achievement. Something that leads to crossing something off your to-do list or a small piece of a task that you've been avoiding. This is building mastery (B).

• Reduce your vulnerability to Emotion Mind by using cope ahead (C) to plan for an upcoming difficult situation and rehearse being skillful. If you're someone who tends to bury your head in the sand and avoid when you know something stressful is heading your way, this is the skill for you to practice as needed.

• Take care of your PLEASE skills as much as possible. No one is expected to be perfect. Instead, determine which of these skills may be most important for you to work on, and make a plan to practice that skill every day. For example, if your sleep is all messed up and you know that this makes you a terror during the day, start taking steps toward better sleep hygiene. If you have stopped exercising and notice that you feel sluggish and bad about yourself as a result, make a plan for getting some form of exercise in your day, no matter how small.

Radical Acceptance (pages 130–133):

• Recognize that any moment of the day provides an opportunity for Radical Acceptance.

• Notice when you might be rejecting reality (your body is tense, you're having lots of judgments) and practice adopting a willing, easy posture. Say things to yourself like "I accept this moment exactly as it is," "everything is as it should be," and "this couldn't be any other way." Take slow, deep breaths in and out as you do so.

Using this book is just the beginning. DBT skills are not miracle cures. We wish we could offer you something that instantly relieved you of all your struggles (bring on the Nobel Prize! And the billions of dollars!). The truth is these skills take intentional and consistent practice to have long-lasting impact. Applying the skills in your everyday life is where the real change happens. There will be setbacks. That's to be expected—those moments are a natural part of the process and of life. What's important is that you continue to practice, notice the impact, and refine. Over time, you'll notice critical differences in how you respond to challenging situations and emotions. We hope these skills bring you greater confidence and self-compassion, and a sense of control in your life.

INDEX

ABOUT THE AUTHORS

Shireen L. Rizvi, PhD, is Professor of Psychiatry and Behavioral Sciences at Montefiore Einstein Medical Center in New York, where she serves as Director of Psychology Training and Director of DBT Services and Research. Dr. Rizvi earned her doctorate under the mentorship of Marsha M. Linehan. She has received extensive grant funding and published dozens of research papers. Dr. Rizvi is board certified in cognitive and behavioral therapies and DBT. Her mission is to get DBT tools to as many people as possible. Her website is *www.shireenrizvi.com.*

Jesse Finkelstein, PsyD, is a clinical psychologist, educator, and creator of innovative DBT-based interventions. He has trained extensively in DBT and other evidence-based treatments, with a specialization in emotion dysregulation, posttraumatic stress disorder, and obsessive–compulsive disorder. Dr. Finkelstein's work bridges clinical practice, research, and creative design to make DBT skills more accessible and engaging. His website is *www.therahive.com.*